Innovative Practice Models for Acute and Critical Care

Guest Editor

MARIA R. SHIREY, PhDc, MS, MBA, RN, NEA-BC, FACHE

CRITICAL CARE NURSING CLINICS OF NORTH AMERICA

www.ccnursing.theclinics.com

Consulting Editor
JANET FOSTER, PhD, RN, CNS, CCRN

December 2008 • Volume 20 • Number 4

SAUNDERS an imprint of ELSEVIER, Inc.

W.B. SAUNDERS COMPANY
A Division of Elsevier Inc.

Elsevier Inc., 1600 John F. Kennedy Blvd., Suite 1800, Philadelphia, PA 19103-2899

http://www.theclinics.com

CRITICAL CARE NURSING CLINICS OF NORTH AMERICA Volume 20, Number 4
December 2008 ISSN 0899-5885, ISBN-13: 978-1-4160-6284-4, ISBN-10: 1-4160-6284-X

Editor: Katie Hartner

Critical Care Nursing Clinics of North America (ISSN 0899-5885) is published quarterly by Elsevier Inc., 360 Park Avenue South, New York, NY 10010-1710. Months of issue are March, June, September, and December. Business and Editorial Offices: 1600 John F. Kennedy Blvd., Suite 1800, Philadelphia, PA19103-2899. Customer Service Office: 6277 Sea Harbor Drive, Orlando, FL 32887-4800. Periodicals postage paid at New York, NY and additional mailing offices. Subscription prices are $130.00 per year for US individuals, $233.00 per year for US institutions, $68.00 per year for US students and residents, $167.00 per year for Canadian individuals, $292.00 per year for Canadian institutions, $191.00 per year for international individuals, $292.00 per year for international institutions and $99.00 per year for Canadian and foreign students/residents. To receive student/resident rate, orders must be accompanied by name of affiliated institution, data of term, and the signature of program/residency coordinator on institution letterhead. Orders will be billed at individual rate until proof of status is received. Foreign air speed delivery is included in all Clinics subscription prices. All prices are subject to change without notice. **POSTMASTER:** Send address changes to Critical Care Nursing Clinics of North America, Elsevier Periodicals Customer Service, 11830 Westline Industrial Drive, St. Louis, MO 63146. **Customer Service: 1-800-654-2452 (US). From outside the United States, call 1-314-453-7041. Fax: 1-314-453-5170. E-mail: JournalsCustomerServiceusa@elsevier.com (for print support) and JournalsOnlineSupport-usa@elsevier.com (for online support).**

Reprints. For copies of 100 or more of articles in this publication, please contact the Commercial Reprints Department, Elsevier Inc., 360 Park Avenue South, New York, New York, 10010-1710; Tel.: (212) 633-3813, Fax: (212) 462-1935, and E-mail: reprints@elsevier.com.

Critical Care Nursing Clinics of North America is covered in *MEDLINE/PubMed (Index Medicus), International Nursing Index, Nursing Citation Index, Cumulative Index to Nursing and Allied Health Literature, and RNdex Top 100.*

Printed in the United States of America.

Contributors

CONSULTING EDITOR

JANET FOSTER, PhD, RN, CNS, CCRN
Assistant Professor, College of Nursing, Texas
Woman's University, Houston, Texas

GUEST EDITOR

**MARIA R. SHIREY, PhDc, MS, MBA,
RN, NEA-BC, FACHE**
Principal, Shirey & Associates, Evansville,
Indiana

AUTHORS

G. RUMAY ALEXANDER, EdD, RN
Associate Clinical Professor, School
of Nursing; and Director, Office of Multicultural
Affairs, University of North Carolina at Chapel
Hill, Chapel Hill, North Carolina

IRMAJEAN BAJNOK, RN, MScN, PhD
Director of International Affairs and Best
Practice Guidelines Programs, Registered
Nurses' Association of Ontario, Toronto,
Ontario, Canada

TAYA BRILEY, RN, BSN, JD
Attorney, Washington State Hospital
Association, Seattle, Washington

GLADYS M. CAMPBELL, RN, MSN
Executive Director, Northwest Organization
of Nurse Executives, Seattle, Washington

CAROL T. COKER, ARNP, MSN, CWOCN
Coordinator of Wound Ostomy Continence
Nursing, Jackson Health System, Miami,
Florida

ANN LYNN DENKER, ARNP, PhD
Magnet Project Director, Jackson Health
System, Miami; Adjunct Professor of Nursing,
University of Miami School of Nursing and
Health Studies, Coral Gables; and Center
for Nursing Excellence, Miami, Florida

JOHN F. DIXON, MSN, RN, NE-BC
Nurse Researcher and Nursing Leadership/
Management Consultant, The Center for
Nursing Education and Research, Baylor
University Medical Center, Dallas, Texas

LISA DONAHUE, DrNP, RN
Director, Inpatient Quality and Innovation,
Patient Care Services, UPMC Shadyside,
Pittsburgh, Pennsylvania

KAREN NEIL DRENKARD, PhD, RN, NEA-BC
Director, Magnet Recognition Program,
American Nurses Credentialing Center, Silver
Spring, Maryland

KATHRYN M. EWERS, RN, BA, MEd
Educator and Project Leader for Evidence-
Based Nursing, Education and Development,
Jackson Health System, Miami; and Adjunct
Faculty, University of Miami School of Nursing
and Health Studies, Coral Gables, Florida

JANET G. FOSTER, RN, PhD
Associate Professor, Texas Woman's
University, College of Nursing, Houston, Texas

JEFFREY T. HUBER, PhD
Associate Professor, Texas Woman's
University, School of Library and Information
Studies, Houston, Texas

PAMELA R. JEFFRIES, DNS, RN, FAAN, ANEF
Associate Professor, Department of Adult Health and Associate Dean for Undergraduate Programs, Indiana University School of Nursing, Indianapolis, Indiana

HEATHER K.S. LASCHINGER, PhD, RN
Distinguished Professor, Associate Dean for Research, University of Western Ontario, School of Nursing, London, Ontario, Canada

MILISA MANOJLOVICH, PhD, RN, CCRN
Assistant Professor, Division of Nursing Business and Health Systems, University of Michigan School of Nursing, Ann Arbor, Michigan

ANGELA M. McNELIS, PhD, RN
Associate Professor, Department of Environments for Health, and Director of Special Projects for the Office of the Associate Dean for Undergraduate Programs, Indiana University School of Nursing, Indianapolis, Indiana

MARY A. MYERS, RN, MSN
Administrative Director, Clarian Inpatient Medicine, Clarian Health, Indianapolis, Indiana

KENNETH PETERSON, MS, MA, RN
Family Nurse Practitioner, Plumley Village Health Services, University of Massachusetts Memorial Medical Center, Worcester; and PhD Candidate, The Heller School for Social Policy and Management, Brandeis University, Waltham, Massachusetts

PATRICIA REID PONTE, RN, DNSc, FAAN
Senior Vice President, Nursing and Patient Care Services, Dana-Farber Cancer Institute; and Director, Oncology Nursing and Clinical Services, Brigham and Women's Hospital, Boston, Massachusetts

SANDRA RADER, RN, MSA
Chief Nursing Officer and Vice President, Patient Care Services, UPMC Shadyside, Pittsburgh, Pennsylvania

KEVIN D. REED, RN, MSN, NE-BC, CPHQ
Director of Clinical Operations, Adult Critical Care Services, Clarian Health, Methodist Hospital, Indianapolis, Indiana; Immediate Past Chair, American Association of Critical Care Nurses Certification Corporation, Aliso Viejo, California

CAROL A. REINECK, PhD, MSN, MEd, RN, FAAN, NEA-BC
Chair and Associate Professor, Department of Acute Nursing Care, The University of Texas Health Science Center at San Antonio School of Nursing, San Antonio, Texas

MARIA R. SHIREY, PhDc, MS, MBA, RN, NEA-BC, FACHE
Principal, Shirey & Associates, Evansville, Indiana

TRUDI B. STAFFORD, RN, PhD
Doctoral Candidate, Texas Woman's University, College of Nursing, Houston, Texas; and Chief Nursing Officer & Vice President of Patient Care Services, University of Pittsburgh Medical Center – Passavant/Passavant Cranberry, Pittsburgh, Pennsylvania

PAMELA KLAUER TRIOLO, PhD, RN, FAAN
Chief Nursing Officer, UPMC, Pittsburgh, Pennsylvania

CORINNE A. WHEELER, PhD, RN
Assistant Professor, Department of Environments for Health, Indiana University School of Nursing, Indianapolis, Indiana

ANNE YOUNG, RN, EdD
Professor, Texas Woman's University, College of Nursing, Houston, Texas

Contents

> This article provides a historical overview of nursing models of care for acute and critical care based on currently available literature. Models of care are defined and their advantages and disadvantages presented. The distinctive differences between care delivery models and professional practice models are explained. The historical overview of care delivery models provides a foundation for the introduction of best practice models that will shape the environment for acute and critical care in the future.

> The purpose of this article is to describe selected best practices in acute and critical care. The evidence base for these models is steadily building. Attributes of past, present, and emerging models are discussed in the context of important considerations such as stress, capacity, and infection. The author offers suggestions for using what we know to advance models of care in the information age that has only just begun.

> The Beacon Award for Critical Care Excellence recognizes individual critical care units that have met rigid criteria for excellence, exhibiting high-quality standards and exceptional care of patients and their families. Used as a framework for quality, the award criteria focus on structure, process, and outcomes that enable quality to emerge in the critical care environment. The journey toward meeting Beacon Award criteria can produce long-lasting changes that transform unit-based culture and lead to sustained excellence.

Evolving Models

Critical Care Nursing Clinics of North America

THE CLINICS ARE NOW AVAILABLE ONLINE!

Access your subscription at:
www.theclinics.com

Preface

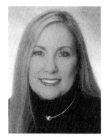

Maria R. Shirey, PhDc, MS, MBA, RN, NEA-BC, FACHE
Guest Editor

The state of health care delivery in America is in need of a major overhaul. In its groundbreaking report, *Crossing the Quality Chasm: A New Health System for the 21st Century,* the Institute of Medicine (IOM) issued a call to action[1] signaling the need for "a fundamental, sweeping redesign of the entire health system".[2] The comprehensive report proposed six aims for fostering innovation and care delivery improvements. According to the IOM report,[1] health care delivery systems should be safe, effective, patient-centered, timely, efficient, and equitable. Concurrent with the six aims, *Crossing the Quality Chasm* also called for information technology system enhancements, quicker translation of research findings into practice, and the development of high-performance health care teams within learning organizations. The care environment[1] was seen as so important to quality and patient safety that, as it's title illustrates, the next landmark IOM report focused exclusively on *Keeping Patients Safe* by transforming the work environment of nurses.[3]

To facilitate the sweeping changes needed to comply with the IOM recommendations in both reports,[1,2] new practice and care delivery models are needed to advance the nation's patient care quality and safety agenda. The goal of this themed issue of *Critical Care Nursing Clinics of North America* is to present innovative practice models that are evidence-based and have been or currently are being implemented in acute and critical care practice environments. The issue contributes toward filling the gap that currently exists between research and practice by illustrating examples of current, evolving, and future models of practice. The current and evolving models presented have been tested and have demonstrated their effectiveness in enriching

the nurse's practice environment and improving patient care outcomes.

OVERVIEW OF CARE DELIVERY MODELS

Shirey opens the issue with a historical overview of care delivery models and provides distinction between care delivery models and professional practice models. The historical overview provides the foundation for introducing the article by Reineck on best practice models that help to create the environment in acute and critical care for the future. Collectively, these two articles provide over half a century of historical perspective on models of care and incorporate context as an important professional practice consideration.

CURRENT MODELS

Reed introduces our readers to the American Association of Critical-Care Nurses (AACN) Beacon Award as a framework for quality and a vehicle for recognizing individual critical care units for excellence. Dixon translates into practice the AACN's standards for establishing and sustaining healthy work environments and provides tools to validate the healthy work environment in professional nursing practice. Drenkard discusses the findings of a quasi-experimental, longitudinal study to reduce work intensity for hospital nurses in order to create a theory-based human caring environment in the acute care workplace of a Magnet-designated health care system. Alexander conveys the importance of intentionality in developing cultural competency and disseminates to a broader audience the American Organization of Nurse Executives guiding principles for diversity in health care organizations. Ewers, Coker,

Crit Care Nurs Clin N Am 20 (2008) xi–xii
doi:10.1016/j.ccell.2008.08.006

Bajnok, and Denker report on their International Center of Excellence partnership with the Registered Nurses Association of Ontario to build evidence-based nursing practice capacity and to introduce a curricular model for increasing the use of best practice guidelines.

EVOLVING MODELS

Myers and Reed familiarize readers with the virtual intensive care unit environment, a redesigned model of care that utilizes state-of-the art technology to enhance patient care quality and safety. Stafford, Myers, Young, Foster, and Huber build the science on telemedicine and discuss the findings of an ethnographic study that describes what it is like to work in the virtual intensive care unit environment. Reid Ponte and Peterson present the Dana Farber Cancer Institute's experience in embracing a patient- and family-centered model of care and a culture of quality and safety. Donahue, Rader, and Triolo showcase the Robert Wood Johnson Foundation's and the Institute of Healthcare Improvement's collaboration in creating the Transforming Care at the Bedside project, and discuss their organization's involvement as a participating facility to nurture care delivery innovation across acute and critical care. Jeffries, McNelis, and Wheeler provide an overview of simulation as a vehicle for enhancing an interdisciplinary collaborative practice model that uses technology to facilitate communication, critical thinking, and problem solving. Manojlovich and Laschinger translate research findings into practice and describe how the Nursing Worklife Model can be applied in acute and critical care to improve the practice environment for nurses and enhance quality outcomes for patients and families.

FUTURE MODELS

Campbell closes the issue with a thought provoking and reflective article that explores the development of future practice models. The author offers suggestions of the desired elements of future practice models and discusses collaborative and interdisciplinary work in progress that provide a transformational and synergistic approach to "bundled redesign" in acute and critical care.

CONCLUSION

The 14 articles in this issue collectively address the IOM recommendations for patient care quality and safety and present innovative models that produce positive outcomes for patients, families, staff, and organizations. In keeping with the journal's North American focus and broad professional nursing representation, the articles showcase the work of clinicians, educators, researchers, and nurses in leadership and management practice from across the United States and Canada.

Maria R. Shirey, PhDc, MS, MBA, RN, NEA-BC, FACHE
Shirey & Associates
10700 Coach Light Drive
Evansville, IN 47725, USA

E-mail address:
mrs@mail2maria.com (M.R. Shirey)

REFERENCES

1. Institute of Medicine. Crossing the Quality Chasm: A New Health System for the 21st Century. Washington, DC: The National Academies Press; 2001.
2. Kimball B, Joynt J, Cherner D, et al. The quest for new innovative care delivery models. J Nurs Adm 2007; 37(9):392–8.
3. Institute of Medicine. Keeping Patients Safe: Transforming the Work Environment of Nurses. Washington, DC: The National Academies Press; 2004.

Nursing Practice Models for Acute and Critical Care: Overview of Care Delivery Models

Maria R. Shirey, PhDc, MS, MBA, RN, NEA-BC, FACHE

KEYWORDS

- Models • Care delivery models
- Professional practice models • Healthy work environment
- Synergy • Acute and critical care

Nursing history is replete with models of care dating back to the turn of the 20th century. From the years of Florence Nightingale to today's information age, models of care, in their pure or blended forms, continue to influence nursing practice in acute and critical care. Although many models of care have been crafted and used, most still lack a strong empirical base. This article provides a historical overview of nursing models of care for acute and critical care based on currently available literature. Models of care are defined and their advantages, disadvantages, and related quality outcomes presented. The distinctive differences between care delivery models and professional practice models are explained. The historical overview of care delivery models provides a foundation for the introduction of best practice models that will shape the environment for future acute and critical care.

OVERVIEW OF CARE DELIVERY MODELS
What are Models of Care?

The term *model* refers to a structural design or representation of which something is to be made.[1] In the context of care delivery models in nursing, this term refers to a framework in which to organize the work of caring for patients.[2] Most care delivery models in nursing are theoretical or conceptual[3] and, over time, many have been tested, enriched, and challenged.[4] There is no right model of care; ultimately, effectiveness determines which care delivery model to use.[5]

Over the course of nursing history, many care delivery models have been used[2] either in their pure forms or as blended models. Implementation of a care delivery model usually reflects the social values, predominant management philosophy, and economic considerations[6] of the times. Industrial, societal, and professional trends also play roles in the selection of a care delivery model for nursing services.

Traditional Care Delivery Models

Table 1 summarizes five care delivery models. Four models are traditional (total patient care, functional nursing, team nursing, primary nursing) and one is contemporary (patient-centered care). Each has its unique configuration, distinct advantages, disadvantages, and related quality outcomes. Although models of care may not be perfect, they are useful[4] and provide a blueprint for change.[3,7]

Total patient care

Total patient care is the oldest model of nursing care delivery and focuses on the complete care (body, mind, and spirit) of each patient.[2] From 1890 to 1929, graduate nurses working as private duty nurses delivered total patient care in the homes of the sick.[8] Using the case method (each patient is a case), each nurse assumed total care for one patient and one patient only. Private duty nurses worked mostly through registries operated by medical and nursing societies or hospitals.

Shirey & Associates, 10700 Coach Light Drive, Evansville, IN 47725, USA
E-mail address: mrs@mail2maria.com

Crit Care Nurs Clin N Am 20 (2008) 365–373
doi:10.1016/j.ccell.2008.08.014
0899-5885/08/$ – see front matter © 2008 Elsevier Inc. All rights reserved.

Table 1
Traditional and contemporary care delivery models

Model	Historical Evolution	Description/Focus	Duration of Care Delivery	Advantages	Disadvantages
Traditional care delivery models					
Total patient care	Oldest model of nursing care delivery; from 1890–1929, graduate nurses worked mostly as private duty nurses outside hospitals; from 1930–1940, Great Depression forced decrease in private duty nursing, graduate nurses returned to hospitals as senior nursing students; since 1980, resurgence in total patient care	From 1890–1929, total patient care conceived as 1:1 nurse–patient relationship using case method model; from 1930–1940, total patient care broadened to more patients assigned to one nurse; since 1980, uses primarily RN staff to deliver care with some support from non-RNs	From 1890–1929, one shift or extended 1:1 patient assignment agreed upon contractually; from 1930–1940, one shift; since 1980, one shift with "shift" definition varying beyond standard 8 h/d	Continuity of care is guaranteed for a given shift; RNs before 1930s were self-employed, had more practice autonomy; patient needs met quickly; close nurse–patient relationship	Continuity of care not guaranteed throughout the hospital stay; high cost of 1:1 RN/patient ratio
Functional nursing	Used from 1940–1960; model became popular during World War II; associated with nursing shortage in United States and in battlefields	Model divides work into tasks assigned to nursing and support personnel; delegation of tasks based on knowledge, skills, and abilities; nurse manager makes all assignments; less RN staff empowerment	One shift	Requires fewer RNs; cost-efficient in short run; division of labor clearly outlined	Fosters fragmentation in care that is not holistic; no one person accountable for total patient care; exposure to many caregivers; focus on tasks over critical thinking, professional autonomy, and personal development

Model	History	Description	Duration	Advantages	Disadvantages
Team nursing	Used from 1950–1960; model emerged following World War II; absorbed military corpsmen into nursing-assistant roles; associated with nursing shortage in United States; addressed problems of functional nursing	Model uses a group of health care workers (RNs, licensed practical nurses, nurse's aides) to deliver care; one RN serves as team leader; focus on collaboration to meet comprehensive needs of a group of patients	One shift; team may care for same patients over the hospital stay	RN has accountability for supervision and coordination of patient care; model incorporates and maximizes skills of both RN and non-RN staff; patients interact with fewer caregivers; care is less fragmented than in functional nursing	Hierarchical model limits professional autonomy; teams require many members; most expensive model; communication among team members is complex and affects efficiencies
Primary nursing	Emerged in 1960s and popular through 1990s; model addresses limitations of previous models; intermittently retained and abandoned by many organizations during re-engineering of the 1990s; since 2000, contemporary version of primary nursing conceptualized as relationship-centered care	Developed to overcome limitations of functional and team nursing with emphasis on the professional aspects of nursing practice; RN is primary nurse assigned to coordinate and deliver total patient care to a group of patients; incorporates associate nurses to deliver care in primary nurse's absence; initially associated with mostly RN staff	24 h/d from admission to discharge	Better incorporates the professional aspects of nursing practice (autonomy, clinical judgment, and decision making); focus on holistic care of patients across the course of a hospitalization; associated with enhanced quality outcomes and more satisfied nurses	Wide variation in implementation; total accountability may be overwhelming to the RN; may be costly in the short run as it requires higher RN complement; intimidating for less skilled RNs

(continued on next page)

Table 1
(continued)

Contemporary care delivery model

Model	Historical Evolution	Description/Focus	Duration of Care Delivery	Advantages	Disadvantages
Patient-centered care (or patient-focused care or expanded to patient–family–centered care)	Model pioneered by Planetree Institute in 1978; gained momentum during re-engineering of the 1990s; improved over time; now recommended by Institute of Medicine[14]; model focuses on patient and family needs	Multidisciplinary services are brought directly to patient; care team members care for a group of patients on a unit; care is standardized with emphasis on adopting best practices; care delivery uses any of the traditional models (alone or in combination); most direct care given by an RN with unit assistive personnel (nurse's aides, technicians); cross-trained personnel in this model perform additional duties; incorporates elements of case management for patient populations to focus on both quality of care and cost containment (use of care maps)	One shift for unit based staff; case management assists in coordination of care across hospital stay	Convenient for patients; expedites care; better incorporates professional practice of various care team members; With emphasis on continuum of care, less fragmentation in care; more efficient use of resources; enhanced teamwork, collaboration, and communication	Success depends on having right staff at right time to meet patient needs; care delivery model is not "pure," making it difficult to articulate the elements of the care delivery model; care model requires RN to be both good clinician and good manager

These nurses either worked one shift or contracted for an extended assignment, often living in the patient's home. Before 1930, most patient care took place in the home rather than in the hospital setting. Hospitals then were staffed primarily by student nurses (unpaid) and a few supervisory graduate nurses.

From 1930 to 1940, the Great Depression led to a decrease in private duty nursing, forcing many nurses to return to hospital employment as senior nursing students in exchange for room and board.[8] The case method continued to be used for patient assignments[6] except that the nurse workload in the hospital increased, making it impossible in most places to maintain the 1:1 nurse-to-patient ratio. In the 1980s, total patient care resurfaced after a long hiatus. Using the total patient care model, a staff made up primarily of registered nurses (RNs) provides complete care that addresses the holistic needs of a group of patients. In some settings with high patient acuity (critical care, labor and delivery), 1:1 nursing still occurs. With total patient care, the individual RN usually receives some level of support from non-RN personnel, such as licensed practical nurses or unit-based nursing assistants or technicians.

According to the literature, "the quality associated with this model is higher than for team and/or functional nursing models, but not as high as in a primary care nursing model."[6] Total patient care in the short run may seem more costly because it requires a high percentage of RNs to deliver care. In the long term, however, total patient care may be more cost- and quality-effective as research increasingly demonstrates that care delivery with a higher RN complement (especially nurses with bachelor of science in nursing degrees) results in enhanced nursing vigilance that translates into improved patient safety and better patient care outcomes.[9]

Functional nursing

Functional nursing is a model of nursing care delivery that became popular during World War II. During that period, many nurses left the country to serve abroad during the war. At the same time, hospitals all across the United States were expanding and looking to add nurses. Supply of nurses in the United States thus fell just at a time when demand for nurses in the United States was rising, creating a shortage.[8] Conceived with industrial mass production in mind, this model uses an assembly-line approach to patient care and maximizes the skills of a varied workforce, not an all-RN staff.[6] The focus of this model is on achieving efficiencies through division of tasks.

Tasks are delegated and assigned based on an individual's skills, knowledge, and abilities. Under this model, RNs may focus on complex patient care needs within their scope of practice while support personnel address routine aspects of patient care. In functional nursing, nurse managers or charge nurses make all assignments; they handle all patient-related reports.[2]

Functional nursing requires fewer RNs and thus may be more cost-efficient in the short run. The model clearly delineates the division of labor and uses skills of a variety of individuals (not just the RN) to provide care for a large number of patients. A disadvantage of functional nursing is that it fragments care and no one person is accountable for total patient care. Given its technical orientation and emphasis on ritual, this model does not encourage professional nursing autonomy or personal development beyond task mastery. The fragmentation of patient care predisposes to thinking in silos ("It's not my job"), impersonal patient care (many individuals performing pieces of total care), errors, and omissions.[6] This fragmentation in care threatens patient safety.

Team nursing

Team nursing is a model of nursing care delivery that emerged after World War II as a way to incorporate military corpsmen into patient care and to address the existing nursing shortage.[2] Corpsmen, who were nonlicensed individuals trained to perform simple care and technical procedures, received on-the-job retraining to function as nursing assistants in hospitals. In team nursing, an RN is the leader of a team that usually consists of other RNs, licensed practical nurses, and nursing assistants. The RN team leader appropriately delegates patient care duties to members of the team and supervises the care for all patients on the team. Each team provides care to a designated group of patients and the team leader usually does not take a patient assignment. This model is hierarchical with reports exchanged between charge nurse and charge nurse, charge nurse and team leader, and team leader and team members.[6] Advantages of team nursing include the use of multilevel personnel and, compared to functional nursing, better continuity of care, fewer caregivers (less functional focus), more RN direction and coordination, and enhanced communication among team members. Quality of care in the team model is reportedly higher than in functional nursing primarily because the RN oversees the function of the team and is responsible for and accountable for fewer patients.[6] A disadvantage of the team model is that it requires allocation of time for communication among team members. If time for such communication is not provided, fragmentation in care occurs. Because team nursing requires more personnel (albeit not all RNs), the costs are not necessarily lower. The team model requires strong RN delegation and supervisory skills, something that, if missing, may undermine effectiveness of the team.

Primary nursing

Primary nursing is a model of nursing care delivery that emerged in the late 1960s to address the limitations of functional and team nursing. The model surfaced at a time when the nursing profession started moving away from task orientation and began focusing more on nursing professionalism and accountability. In primary nursing, a staff nurse serves as primary nurse and in this role is assigned care coordination responsibility for three to four patients from admission to discharge.[10] For the duration of the hospitalization, the primary nurse has 24-hour-per-day accountability for planning, delivering, monitoring, and coordinating care for those patients. When the primary nurse is not actually providing patient care, an associate nurse delivers the care following the primary nurse's care plan. Assignments in primary nursing are based on patient need and staff abilities. Decision making in this model is decentralized and occurs close to the bedside.

The major advantage of primary nursing is enhanced continuity of care, improved quality of care, and empowerment of professional nursing practice. Care delivery under a primary nursing model is holistic and patient-focused. Development of a trusting nurse–patient relationship is therapeutic for both patients and nurses. Under this model, the professional aspects of nursing practice, including autonomy, clinical judgment, and decision making are maximized. A disadvantage of primary nursing is that its implementation may vary from organization to organization, yielding different results. The model is sensitive to nurse-to-patient ratios and is difficult to implement when RNs are assigned too many patients. The 24-hour RN accountability, a hallmark of the model, may be overwhelming to many nurses.

Although primary nursing came to be associated with an all-RN staff,[5] implementation of this model does not necessarily require an all-RN staff.[11] In the 1970s, the use of this model of care expanded rapidly. However, due to hospital cost containment efforts of the 1980s and early 1990s, the model was eliminated in many institutions. Primary nursing has resurfaced today configured as relationship-centered care.[12]

Contemporary Care Delivery Model: Patient-Centered Care

Table 1 summarizes the elements of patient-centered care (also called patient-focused care or expanded as patient-family–centered care),[13] a more contemporary care delivery model that incorporates a multidisciplinary approach. In this model, the necessary services for patient care are brought to the patient. The model is decentralized and, in its highest evolution, all needed services for a given population (radiology, pharmacy, laboratory, physical therapy) are available at the point of care or in very close geographic proximity[2] to the patient. Staffing decisions are made based on patient care needs and actual care delivery uses any of the traditional models alone or in combination. An RN provides most of the direct patient care with other personnel (nursing assistants or patient care technicians) assisting. Individuals cross-trained to perform additional duties make up multidisciplinary care teams and collaborate to address patient and family needs. Incorporation of case managers into this model helps address coordination of care across hospitalizations and assists in ensuring high quality of care and control of costs.

Advantages of patient-centered care include enhanced convenience and more expeditious care to patients and families. The model is highly customized to meet patient wants, needs, and preferences[14] and more actively engages both patients and families in care processes.[15] Patient-centered care facilitates interdisciplinary communication, collaboration, and coordination to better facilitate smooth transitions across the care continuum.[14] In this model, care is standardized through use of care maps and emphasis is given to controlling patient care costs and use of resources. A major disadvantage of the model is that in many institutions, implementation of patient-centered care resulted in cutting hospital costs through reduction of RN staff.[2] Increasing workload for hospital nurses without concomitant increases in resources threatens nurse-sensitive outcomes and has been linked to a decline in patient safety.[16] Because there is not one standard definition of patient-centered care and it may incorporate a variety of care delivery models, patient-centered care is poorly understood[15] and difficult for many nurses to articulate.

Future Care Delivery Models

As the health care industry continues to evolve, so will the care delivery models used in acute and critical care. A thorough discussion of future care delivery models is beyond the scope of this article.

Those designing such models should avail themselves of pertinent decision-making data, evaluation criteria,[17] and useful guiding frameworks. One such framework, the American Association of Nurse Executives' Guiding Principles for Future Patient Care Delivery,[18] offers assistance in crafting those models. Regardless of their configuration, future care delivery models "should be in strategic alignment with the organization, sustainable over time, and replicable."[3] These models should address structure, process, and outcomes that focus on patient safety, quality, and cost containment.

PROFESSIONAL PRACTICE MODELS

A professional practice model (PPM) describes how a professional practice environment is created.[3] A PPM serves as a framework for guiding and aligning clinical practice, education, administration, and research.[19] PPMs have five subsystems: professional values, professional relationships, a care delivery model, management or governance, and professional recognition and rewards.[3,20]

Professional values constitute the guiding beliefs that form the core of professional practice. These beliefs are made visible in a nursing philosophy statement that incorporates the organizational mission and vision and is supported by a theoretical foundation that is a good organizational fit.

Professional relationships describe interactions that occur among nurses and with members of other disciplines when providing patient care services. These relationships ideally should be respectful, patient-centered, conducive to interdisciplinary collaboration, and outcomes oriented.

The care delivery model as previously discussed consists of identifying traditional or contemporary models within the PPM. Selection of the care delivery model should be consistent with the other subsystems in the PPM.

Management or governance within the PPM specifies the structures and processes that will be used for decision making related to unit and organizational operations. Most governance structures today are decentralized and participative (shared decision-making as compared with hierarchical and prescriptive approaches) and many reflect the structural empowerment tenets of the Magnet Recognition Program.[21]

Professional recognition and rewards address the systems in place to compensate nurses for their work and to recognize their contributions to patient, organizational, and professional outcomes. Pay for nurses has historically been hourly. However, many incentive compensation methods in use reward nurses for their individual contributions (career ladders) and for their ability to collaborate as team members to reach organizational targets (operating margin, employee turnover) and patient care targets (patient satisfaction, performance on nurse sensitive indicators). Underlying most recognition and reward programs is accountability for professional performance and pride in professional practice.

Many PPMs are in use today in acute and critical care environments throughout the country. One example of a PPM is the American Association of Critical-Care Nurses' Synergy Model,[22] which is in use at Clarian Health in Indianapolis,[23,24] where it serves the dual purposes of providing a framework for patient care delivery and also for elevating professional nursing practice. Another PPM easily accessible on the Internet[25] and unique for its focus on interdisciplinary practice is the one at Massachusetts General Hospital in Boston.[19] Although these two models represent only a tiny sampling of the PPM universe, they nevertheless provide helpful examples that capture the essence of PPMs.

CARE DELIVERY MODELS VERSUS PROFESSIONAL PRACTICE MODELS
Distinction

Although the terms care delivery model and PPM are often used interchangeably, they are not synonymous.[3,26] Care delivery models focus on how care is structurally organized to facilitate nursing work and quality outcomes.[17] PPMs, on the other hand, address how nurses are supported in delivering care. The identification and design of the PPM within the nursing services department should come first; this careful decision should then drive the selection of a care delivery model. A care delivery model is only one piece of a PPM, which in turn supports a professional practice environment.[3]

Other factors, such as economic, regulatory, and workforce considerations (especially skill mix), play roles in the selection of the care delivery model. Under a scenario of constraints, however, the best care delivery model should be selected given the PPM chosen and the desire to do what is right for patients, families, and organizations. Each organization's unique requirements (especially at the unit level) should guide the development of the preferred care delivery model.[17]

Application

The philosophy of nursing, values, and desired patient care and organizational outcomes guide the selection of the care delivery model in a given organization. For example, a hypothetical organization that places great emphasis on compassionate care may develop a written philosophy of nursing that is based on caring science[27] and one that focuses on the humanistic values of caring,[28,29] love, respect, integrity, and well-being. The desired patient care outcomes of the professional practice model would likely be high levels of patient satisfaction, positive healing outcomes (absent or low infection rates), patient safety (absent or low patient falls and medication errors), trust within organizational members, and low employee turnover. To achieve these patient and organizational outcomes while incorporating a caring philosophy, this nursing service would likely select a contemporary care delivery model (patient-centered care or relationship-centered care) while simultaneously building a healthful practice environment.[30,31] To remain consistent with the underlying caring philosophy, both the care delivery model and the PPM would emphasize leadership congruence.[32,33] That is, individuals at all levels of the organization would be expected to show caring, love, respect, and integrity in all decision making such that consideration for the well-being of patients, employees, units, and organizations stays consistently at the forefront of all decisions.

SUMMARY

Care delivery models, their uses, advantages, and disadvantages guide model development for the future. Although no care delivery model is perfect, past models provide an opportunity to learn from experiences and to create a blueprint for change. Ultimately, each organization's unique values and requirements direct the design of the preferred care delivery model within the full PPM. The care delivery model and the other elements of the PPM provide support for the desired professional practice environment.

REFERENCES

1. Merriam-Webster Online Dictionary. Model 2008; Available at: http://www.merriam-webster.com/dictionary/model. Accessed May 30, 2008.
2. Bernat A, Fisher ML. Effective staffing. In: Kelly P, editor. Nursing leadership and management. Clifton Park (NY): Thomson Delmar Learning; 2008. p. 316–39.
3. Wolf GA, Greenhouse PK. Blueprint for design: creating models that direct change. J Nurs Adm 2007;37(9):381–7.
4. Reineck C. Nursing models: a closer look. J Nurs Adm 2007;37(5):209–11.
5. Huber D. Leadership and nursing care management. 3rd edition. Philadelphia: Elsevier Saunders; 2005.
6. Tiedman ME, Lookinland S. Traditional models of care delivery: what have we learned? J Nurs Adm 2004;34(6):291–7.
7. Reineck C. Models of change. J Nurs Adm 2007; 37(9):388–91.
8. Schorr T. 100 years of American nursing: celebrating a century of caring. Philadelphia: Lippincott; 1999.
9. Aiken LH, Clarke SP, Cheung RB, et al. Education levels of hospital nurses and surgical patient mortality. JAMA 2003;290(12):1617–23.
10. Manthey M. An expert answers common questions about primary nursing. Nurs Manage 1973;20(3): 22–4.
11. Manthey M. Primary nursing is alive and well. Am J Nurs 1989;73(1):83–7.
12. Manthey M. aka primary nursing. J Nurs Adm 2003; 33(7/8):369–70.
13. Planetree Institute. Planetree components. 1978. Available at: http://www.planetree.org/about/components.html. Accessed May 30, 2008.
14. Committee on Quality Health Care in America, Institute of Medicine. Crossing the quality chasm: a new health system for the 21st century. Washington, DC: National Academies Press; 2000.
15. Kelleher S. Providing patient-centered care in an intensive care unit. Nurs Stand 2006;21(13): 35–40.
16. Page A, editor. Keeping patients safe: transforming the work environment of nurses. Washington, DC: National Academies Press; 2004.
17. Deutschendorf AL. From past paradigms to future frontiers. J Nurs Adm 2003;33(1):52–9.
18. American Organization of Nurse Executives. AONE guiding principles for future patient care delivery toolkit. 2005. Available at: http://www.aone.org/aone/resource/guidingprinciples.html. Accessed May 30, 2008.
19. Ives Erickson J, Ditomassi M. Professional practice model. In: Feldman HR, editor. Nursing leadership: a concise encyclopedia. New York: Springer Publishing; 2008. p. 457–70.
20. Hoffart N, Woods CQ. Elements of a nursing professional practice model. J Prof Nurs 1996;12(6): 354–64.
21. American Nurses Credentialing Center. Announcing a new model for ANCC's Magnet Recognition Program. 2008. Available at: http://www.nursecredentialing.org/model/index.htm. Accessed May 30, 2008.
22. Kaplow R. AACN synergy model for patient care: a framework to optimize outcomes. Crit Care Nurse 2003;(Suppl):27–30.
23. Kerfoot K. Multihospital system adapts AACN synergy model. Crit Care Nurse 2003;23(5):88–91.
24. Kaplow R, Reed K. The AACN Synergy Model for patient care: a nursing model as a force of magnetism. Nurs Econ 2008;2(1):17–25.

25. Massuchusetts General Hospital. Patient care services professional practice model. 2008. Available at: http://www.massgeneral.org/pcs/abt_prof. asp. Accessed May 30, 2008.

26. Storey S, Linden E, Fisher ML. Showcasing leadership exemplars to propel professional practice model implementation. J Nurs Adm 2008;38(3):138–42.

27. Watson J. Nursing: the philosophy and science of caring. Boulder (CO): University Press; 1985.

28. Boykin A, Schoenhofer S. The role of nursing leadership in creating caring environments in health care delivery systems. Nurs Adm Q 2001;25(3):1–7.

29. Boykin A, Schoenhofer S, Smith N, et al. Transforming practice using a caring-based nursing model. Nurs Adm Q 2003;27(3):223–30.

30. American Association of Critical-Care Nurses. AACN standards for establishing and sustaining healthy work environments: a journey to excellence. Am J Crit Care 2005;14(3):187–97.

31. American Organization of Nurse Executives. AONE principles and elements of a healthful practice/work environment. 2004. Available at: http://www.aone. org/aone/pdf/PrinciplesandElementsHealthfulWork Practice.pdf. Accessed May 30, 2008.

32. Shirey MR. Ethical climate in nursing practice: the leader's role. JONAS Healthc Law Ethics Regul 2005;7(2):59–67.

33. Shirey MR. Authentic leaders creating healthy work environments for nursing practice. Am J Crit Care 2006;15(3):256–67.

Best Practice Models for Acute and Critical Care: Today and into the Future

Carol A. Reineck, PhD, MSN, MEd, RN, FAAN, NEA-BC

KEYWORDS

- Beacon award • Models • Best practices
- Healthy practice environment • Capacity building
- Elders • Evidence-based practice • Synergy
- Interdisciplinary • Collaboration • Team • Stress
- Infection • Innovation • Technology

Acute and critical care nursing today are not constrained by physical boundaries. From high technology settings in metropolitan areas to deployable hospitals in war or disaster zones, we can observe best practices in adult acute and critical care. Where have we come from? Where are we going? Selected past and present models help answer those key questions. In addition, change models, trends for the future, and contextual factors including stress, capacity, and infection are pervasive and bear serious consideration. Nurses and colleagues in caring will use known best practices to help sustain the ongoing development of new models of care to keep patients—and staff—safe. This article describes such selected best practice models for acute and critical care.

LEGACY MEDICAL MODELS OF CARE

More than a decade ago, when critical care models were discussed in the literature, it was not uncommon for them to be expressed simply in terms of the organizational arrangement of physician involvement. For example, models of care in 1995 were described as full-time intensivist (23.1%), consultant (13.7%), multiple consultants (45.6%), or single physician (14.2%).[1] Fortunately,

in that same era, the Society of Critical Care Medicine and the American Association of Critical Care Nurses (AACN) advocated multidisciplinary approach to practice in intensive care units (ICUs). The emphasis was on collaboration and shared responsibility.[2]

This early interprofessional approach[3] for acute and critical care had five characteristics: (1) medical and nursing directors with authority and coresponsibility for ICU management; (2) nursing, respiratory therapy, and pharmacy collaboration with medical staff in a team approach; (3) use of standards, protocols, and guidelines to assure consistent approach to medical, nursing, and technical issues; (4) dedication to coordination and communication for all aspects of ICU management; and (5) emphasis on practitioner certification, research, education, ethical issues, and patient advocacy.

These attributes suggested elements of a best practice model for critical care in the 1990s that are still relevant today: a team approach wherein mortality is minimized, efficiency is optimized, and dignity and compassion for the patient are preserved.[1] The AACN Beacon Award[4] builds on these early best practices. **Table 1** summarizes attributes of best practices in the past, present, and future.

Department of Acute Nursing Care, The University of Texas Health Science Center at San Antonio School of Nursing, 7703 Floyd Curl Drive, Mail Code 7975, San Antonio, TX 78229, USA
E-mail address: reineck@uthscsa.edu

Crit Care Nurs Clin N Am 20 (2008) 375–381
doi:10.1016/j.ccell.2008.08.015

CONTEMPORARY BEST PRACTICES
Acute and Critical Care Excellence and Healthy Work Environments

The AACN Beacon Award Program[4] promotes healthy work environments in ICUs. Areas of impact in the program, found in a helpful audit tool, include recruitment and retention; education, training, and mentoring; evidence-based practice and research; patient outcomes; healing environment; and leadership/organizational ethics. Criteria for receiving a Beacon Award include recognized excellence in the intensive care environments in which nurses work and critically ill patients are cared for; recognized excellence of the highest quality measures, processes, structures, and outcomes based on evidence; recognized excellence in collaboration, communication, and partnerships that support the value of healing and humane environments; and developing a program that contributes to the actualization of AACN's mission, vision, and values.

Studies have shown that units achieving Beacon Award status rate higher on key indicators related to nursing satisfaction, quality of care, leadership, and work environment; in addition, this award allows units to measure their systems, outcomes, and environment against evidence-based criteria.[4] In 2008, 19 critical care units were recognized with the Beacon Award. The Beacon Award is a gold standard, but other models have also been helpful.

One such model, from the American Organization of Nurse Executives (AONE),[5] outlines key organizational success factors for healthy work environments. These include leadership development and effectiveness; empowered collaborative decision-making; work design and service delivery innovation; values-driven organizational culture; recognition and reward systems; and professional growth and accountability.[5] Regional examples of initiatives in acute and critical care to create a healthy work environment include (1) using a participatory planning process to engage managers and staff in revising nursing roles (North Mississippi Medical Center, Tupelo, MS); (2) establishing multidisciplinary collaborative management teams as the foundation of patient-focused care (Hartford Hospital, Hartford, CT); increasing capacity through the "Be a Bed Ahead" program, designed by a multidisciplinary team (Inova Fairfax Hospital, Falls Church, VA); and developing shared governance and multidisciplinary care teams (St. Luke's Regional Medical Center, Boise, ID).[5]

Table 1
Attributes of best practices in acute and critical care: legacy, present, emerging, and future

Legacy Models: 1950–1990	Present and Emerging: 1990–2010	Future: 2010 and Beyond
Organizational arrangement of physician involvement	AACN Beacon Award Program[4]	AACN Beacon Award Program[4]
Collaboration	AACN Synergy Model for Patient Care[7]	AACN Synergy Model for Patient Care[7]
	AACN's standards for establishing and maintaining healthy work environments[7]	AACN's standards for establishing and maintaining healthy work environments[7]
Shared responsibility	AONE Principles and Elements of a Healthful Practice/Work Environment[5]	AONE Principles and Elements of a Healthful Practice/Work Environment[5]
	Clinical Nursing Leadership Learning and Action Progess[6]	Clinical Nursing Leadership Learning and Action Progess[6]
	ACESTAR Model of Knowledge Transformation[13]	ACESTAR Model of Knowledge Transformation[13]
	Nurses Improving Care for the Hospitalized Elderly[11,12]	Nurses Improving Care for the Hospitalized Elderly[11,12]
		Considerations of factors including stress,[16] capacity,[16,17] and infection[4,18]
		Innovative care models[21]
		Infrastructure for innovation[22] and technology[23]

AONE's nine classic principles and elements of a healthful practice/work environment were developed by consensus. They are: (1) collaborative practice culture; (2) communication-rich culture; (3) culture of accountability; (4) presence of adequate numbers of qualified nurses; (5) presence of expert, competent, credible, visible leadership; (6) shared decision-making at all levels; (7) encouragement of professional practice and continued growth/development; (8) recognition of the value of nursing's contribution; and (9) recognition by nurses for their meaningful contribution to practice.[5]

CAPACITY BUILDING AND CAPABILITY DEVELOPMENT

Although healthy work environments lead to positive outcomes for nurses, patients, and organizations, additional positive benefits exist, including capacity building and capability development. Capacity building[6] is an essential process for the survival of any individual or organization. "Capacity itself is the sum of total processes, values and climate within the organization."[6] Capacity building leads to capability development. Capability development, then, is a broader idea. It includes "an emphasis on the overall system, environment, or context within which individuals, organizations, and societies operate and interact."[6] Models not only serve as a guiding light for improving the present situation in acute and critical care, but enhance the capacity to influence operations outside the setting itself.

MODELS FOR PATIENT CARE
Clinical Nursing Leadership Learning and Action Process Model

The Clinical Nursing Leadership Learning and Action Process (CLINLAP) Model in the United Kingdom is a concise and practical way to help manage change within a turbulent environment (eg, acute and critical care). Key attributes are stakeholder mapping and management. CLINLAP essentially includes four phases: (1) service issue analysis; (2) service issue solution formulation; (3) challenging rigid concepts and obsolete assumptions in practice; and (4) focus on agreement by stakeholders.[6]

American Association of Critical Care Nurses Synergy Model for Patient Care

The AACN Synergy Model for Patient Care[7] values patient-centered care. The model demonstrates that positive patient outcomes are achieved when the competencies of the nurse and the characteristics of the patient are matched to meet the needs of the patient. The model guided practice in a military ICU in Iraq.[8] Four aspects of this exceptional model were especially powerful in this austere patient care environment: (1) advocacy and moral agency (a nurse competency); (2) vulnerability (a patient characteristic); (3) response to diversity (a nurse competency); and (4) participation in care (a patient characteristic). Models are portable and useful in nontraditional settings such as mobile hospitals.[8]

MODELS PROMOTE CHANGE

At times, models merge to form a roadmap for change. The AACN and the American College of Chest Physicians (ACCP) merged their respective models. This joint project paved the way for interdisciplinary, patient-focused care.[9] The AACN's six standards for establishing and maintaining healthy work environments are skilled communication, true collaboration, effective decision-making, appropriate staffing, meaningful recognition, and authentic leadership. Each standard is considered essential and requisite to achieving three goals: retention and recruitment, improved job satisfaction, and improved patient and family outcomes. The ACCP endorses the AACN standards and advocates initiatives such as joint physician and nursing education models, interdisciplinary rounds, patient-focused care, challenging the process, and situation–background–assessment–recommendation communication, to name a few (**Fig. 1**).[9]

Critical care is no longer a "place" ... but rather the presence of a collaborative, interdisciplinary and patient-focused approach.[9]

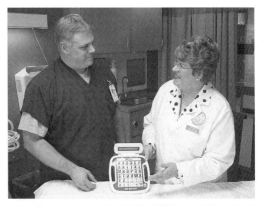

Fig. 1. Charles Reed, RN, MSN, CCRN, and Carol Reineck, RN, PhD, discussing an evidence-based improvement in care for intubated patients and their nurses (Surgical-Trauma Intensive Care Unit, University Hospital, San Antonio, Texas).

Critical care is indeed no longer just a "place." The much-respected legacy of a critical care unit as a "place" has roots in specialized care units for polio patients in the 1950s and early post-anesthesia and coronary care units in the 1970s.[10] Critical care nursing has undergone several phases of development and continues to evolve.

The specialty began with the notion of high-intensity, specialized nursing care, physically set apart from—or in some cases, adjoining—other nursing areas. The physical separation led to ever-increasing specialization. Specialization progressed through development of distinctive areas for the critical care of cardiovascular, surgical, medical, neurologic, neurosurgical, trauma, transplantation, oncology, burn, pediatric, aeromedical, and neonatal patients. Certification programs were a natural and necessary outgrowth of specialization. Today, six decades after inception, critical care is defined as "caring for critically ill patients regardless of the patient's location in the system through a system-wide virtual department that uses a collaborative, interdisciplinary, and patient-focused approach."[9]

TRENDS FOR THE FUTURE
Improved Care of the Hospitalized Elderly

An exceptionally useful model for changing the quality of care delivered to elderly patients is embodied in the work of Nurses Improving Care to Health System Elders (NICHE), funded by the John A. Hartford Foundation.[11] Patients 65 years and older make up 46% of patients in critical care.[11] Few of the nation's 5747 hospitals are prepared to respond to the needs of this vulnerable population. Nearing two decades in its maturity, the NICHE model includes an introduction to NICHE principles and tools through a 2-day leadership conference and identification of a dedicated NICHE coordinator. The tool kit includes the Geriatric Institutional Assessment Profile, four nursing care models, best practice protocols, and educational materials (including gerontologic nursing certification preparation) that supplement the models and protocols. The four nursing care models promoted by NICHE include the Geriatric Resource Nurse Model, the Geriatric Syndrome Management Model, the Acute Care for the Elderly model, and the Comprehensive Discharge Planning/Quality Cost Model of Transitional Care.[11] The Academy of Medical-Surgical Nurses,[12] in collaboration with the Hartford Institute for Geriatric Nursing, created ConsultGeriRN.org as an evidence-based online resource to further the work of NICHE.

CHANGE TO EVIDENCE-BASED PRACTICE

Entire doctoral dissertations have been written on the process of changing the practice environment to one that is evidence-based.[13] The ACESTAR Model of Knowledge Transformation was developed to help drive practice change through evidence.[14] Configured as a simple five-point star, the model explains how knowledge is transformed at five major stages, from original research through the stages of evidence summary, translation, implementation, and evaluation. This model places nursing's previous scientific work within the context of evidence-based practice (EBP) and is proving useful for examining the EBP process, roles in EBP, and research methods to investigate.[14]

In addition to the five-point star, another model for changing to evidence-based practice outlines six steps:

1. assess the need for change in practice;
2. link the problem with interventions and outcomes;
3. synthesize the best evidence;
4. design a change in practice;
5. implement and evaluate the practice change; and
6. integrate and maintain the practice change.[15]

What is the evidence, then, concerning a healthy work environment? The internationally acclaimed, Australia-based Joanna Briggs Institute, in concert with Canadian nurse researchers and practitioners,[16] conducted a comprehensive systematic review focused on the evidence relating to a healthy work environment. In their review of 1275 studies, they culled 57 quantitative and qualitative papers focused on the relationship between teamwork and a healthy work environment. Findings applicable to teamwork in acute and critical care suggested that (1) team functioning can be improved by involving staff (grade of recommendation M2); (2) a multidisciplinary approach results in improved outcomes (grade of recommendation E2); and (3) characteristics of teamwork that promote positive outcomes include accountability, commitment, enthusiasm, motivation, social support, the reduction of conflict, and effective communication (grade of recommendation M2). Grades of recommendations are based on the FAME (Feasibility, Appropriateness, Meaningfulness, and Effectiveness) scale. Grade M2 signifies the evidence provides a moderate rationale for practice change. Grade E2 denotes the effectiveness established to a degree that merits application.[16]

CONSIDERATION OF STRESS, CAPACITY, AND INFECTION

Models for acute and critical care come to life in the context of many dynamic factors, not the least of which include stress, capacity, and infection. Each of these factors alone presents a significant impact on the need for models of care to lead to positive outcomes. Fortunately, investigators[17–19] are advancing knowledge of these contextual factors.

Three Sources of Stress

Models of care in acute and critical care should be designed to help units withstand stress. Stress originates from many sources.[17] Health care delivery systems experience three major stresses: flow stress, clinical stress, and variability in professional abilities and competing responsibilities. Flow stress occurs when patients present for care on a variable basis. Clinical stress emanates from the intensity of the patient's disease state or the intensity of the need for care. The third source of stress, variability in professional abilities and competing responsibilities, refers to staff who function in many roles such as caregiver, preceptor, and charge nurse simultaneously. "If resources are insufficient to tolerate the three stresses…then more medical errors will result."[17]

One strategy for minimizing these stressors is to design models of care that minimize flow stress, clinical stress, and variability in professional abilities and competing responsibilities. An example would be a care delivery model in which volatility in the demand for care is minimized and in which staff have roles that are manageable and appropriate for their abilities and resources. Queing theory[18] can potentiate the process in such a model.

Using Queuing Theory to Boost Capacity

Queuing theory has been applied to predict patient flow,[18] an ever-present issue where acute and critical care are delivered. Queuing theory is widely used for modeling and analysis of processes that involve waiting lines. The investigators studied daily admission rates, length of stay, and the number of available beds in the system. The system was the medical–surgical ICU of an 18-bed, urban children's hospital during a 2-year period. Authors offered four implications for practice:

1. The realistic capacity of an ICU is often significantly overestimated by measures (eg, census) that fail to account for variability of demand.
2. For a system to respond adequately to natural peaks in demand, a predictable number of empty beds must always be ready.
3. Both staffing shortfalls and the presence of patients with lengthy stays need to be considered to appropriately predict the available beds.
4. More effective management of elective surgery scheduling could result in smoother patterns of patient arrival to more carefully conserve expensive and often saturated ICU resources.[18]

The Beacon Award Program's Role in Preventing Infection

Sepsis is the leading cause of death in noncardiac ICUs.[19] The Institute of Medicine[20] identified infection prevention as a key component of patient safety. It is imperative that models of care be designed to minimize this growing and costly threat. Simple handwashing is powerful in preventing infection, yet compliance with handwashing by health care workers is abysmal.[19] Aspects of infection control that should be integrated into models of care would include implementing system-wide organizational awareness, setting high expectations, and providing toolkits. Multiprofessional teams are critical for input and buy-in.

Models of care take on an organized, team-based, educational, and supportive role to reduce infections that affect 750,000 patients who develop severe sepsis as an ultimate complication of infection each year.[19] For example, the AACN's Beacon Award Program standards for adult ICUs[4] call for urinary tract infection rates of <5.6/1000 device days, central line infections of <1.6/1000 device days, decubitus ulcers of <3.7/1000 patient days, and ventilator-associated pneumonia rates of <5.8/1000 patient days. Models that drive standards for outcomes potentially sensitive to nursing (eg, infections) are critical.

KNOWING WHAT WE KNOW, WHERE SHOULD WE GO?

Critical care will celebrate its centennial in the vicinity of the year 2050, 100 years after the first polio units were established in the 1950s. What have we learned to date in the nearly 60 years of caring for critically ill patients and their families in hospitals? We know that early models were focused on physician arrangements. We have learned that contemporary models focus on healthy work environments, leading change, managing complexity, and improving hospital care for vulnerable populations such as the elderly in the context of factors such as stress, capacity, and infection.

The next steps to realize the full potential of models in acute and critical care are to (1) learn about and adopt/adapt existing useful models developed by national professional organizations and foundations; (2) develop and use baseline assessments of practice and care environments; (3) develop and use evidence-based protocols; and (4) consider theory-driven care.[21] Private foundation funding has made it possible for the development of 24 emerging models.[22]

Adding to the profound challenge already described, models of acute and critical care must also consider the importance of infrastructure for innovation[23] in the information age that has only just begun. For example, the American Academy of Nursing's technology drill-down initiative[24] revealed serious defects in that infrastructure, including problems with system and equipment interoperability and the omission of nurse input into technology purchasing decisions. Well-designed future care models and best practices will aim to overcome these and other challenges.

SUMMARY

Spanning six decades, best practices in acute and critical care have steadily evolved from early structural arrangements to contemporary models. Current models focus on culture, environment, evidence, patient-centeredness, and outcomes for both staff and patients. Acute and critical care is no longer a place; rather, it is unconstrained by location. The care is characacterized by a patient-centered, interdisciplinary and collaborative approach.

Care models designed to propel change were described. These included a model to improve the care of the hospitalized elderly and models to help control stress, optimize capacity, and prevent infection. Effective models are those with the aforementioned attributes that, at the same time, encourage ongoing performance improvement in a respectful, communication-rich culture to keep patients—and acute and critical care staff—safe.

REFERENCES

1. Brilli R, Spevetz A, Branson R, et al. Critical care delivery in the intensive care unit: defining clinical roles and the best practice model. Crit Care Med 2001; 29(10):2007–19.
2. Joint position statement: essential provisions for critical care in health system reform. Crit Care Med 1994;22:2017–9.
3. Carlson RW, Weiland D, Wrivathsan K. Does a full-time 24-hour intensivist improve care and efficiency? Crit Care Clin 1996;12:525–51.
4. American Association of Critical Care Nurses (AACN) Beacon Award Program. Available at: http://www.aacn.org.
5. American Organization of Nurse Executives (AONE) and McManis & Monsalve Associates. Healthy Work Environments: Striving for Excellence, vol II, 2003.
6. Alleyne J, Jumaa M. Building the capacity for evidence-based clinical nursing leadership: the role of executive co-coaching and group clinical supervision for quality patient services. J Nurs Manag 2007;15:230–43.
7. American Association of Critical Care Nurses. The AACN synergy model for patient care. Available at: http://www.certcorp.org. Accessed 21 April, 2008.
8. Freyling M, Kesten K, Heath J. The synergy model at work in a military ICU in Iraq. Crit Care Nurs Clin North Am 2008;20:23–9.
9. McCauley K, Irwin R. Changing the work environment in intensive care units to achieve patient-focused care: the time has come. Am J Crit Care 2006;15(6):541–8.
10. Sole ML, Lamborn L, Hartshorn JC. Introduction to critical care nursing. Philadelphia: W.B. Saunders Co; 2001. p. 3.
11. Mezey M, Kobayashi M, Grossman S, et al. Nurses improving care to health system elders (NICHE): Implementation of best practice models. J Nurs Adm 2004;34(10):451–7.
12. Academy of Medical-Surgical Nurses. ConsultGeriRN.org. Available at: http://www.consultgerirn.org. Accessed 14 June, 2008.
13. Clutter, P. The association of factors relating to the registered nurses' uptake of evidence-based clinical practice guidelines in the veterans health administration setting. San Antonio (TX): The University of Texas Health Science Center at San Antonio Graduate School of the Biomedical Sciences, 2007.
14. Academic Center for Evidence-Based Practice (ACE) ACESTAR Model of Knowledge Transformation. Available at: http://www.acestar.uthscsa.edu. Accessed 20 April, 2008.
15. Rosswurm M, Larrabee J. A model for change to evidence-based practice. Image J Nurs Sch 1999; 31:317–22.
16. Pearson A, Porritt K, Doran D, et al. A comprehensive systematic review of evidence on the structure, process, characteristics, and composition of a nursing team that fosters a healthy work environment. Int J Evid Base Healthc 2006;4:118–59.
17. Litvak E, Buerhaus P, Davidoff F, et al. Managing unnecessary variability in patient demand to reduce nursing stress and improve patient safety. Jt Comm J Qual Patient Saf 2005;31(6):330–8.
18. McManus M, Long M, Cooper A, et al. Queuing theory accurately models the need for critical care resources. Anesthesiology 2004;100(5):1271–6.
19. Aragon D, Sole ML. Implementing best practice strategies to prevent infection in the ICU. Crit Care Nurs Clin North Am 2006;18:441–52.
20. Kohn L, Corrigan J, Donaldson M. To err is human: building a safer health system. Washington, DC: National Academy Press; 2000.

21. Pipe T. Optimizing nursing care by integrating theory-driven evidence-based practice. J Nurs Care Qual 2007;22(3):234–8.

22. Robert Wood Johnson Foundation. Innovative care models. Available at: http://www.innovativecaremodels.com. Accessed 14 June, 2008.

23. Porter-O'Grady T. Creating an innovative nursing organization. The voice of nursing leadership: American organization of nurse executives 2008;2(6):6–7.

24. The American Academy of Nursing Commission on Workforce. Technology Drill-down. Available at: http://www.aannet.org.

The American Association of Critical Care Nurse's Beacon Award: A Framework for Quality

Kevin D. Reed, RN, MSN, NE-BC, CPHQ[a,b,*]

KEYWORDS

- Beacon award • Quality • Critical care unit
- Excellence • Healthy work environment

A new health care system for the twenty-first century is beginning to emerge. Catalyzed by two landmark reports from the Institute of Medicine entitled *To Err is Human: Building a Safer Healthcare System*[1] and *Crossing the Quality Chasm: A New Healthcare System for the 21st Century*,[2] a new paradigm for quality and safety has given rise to increased accountability for health care organizations. Nowhere has the impact of this new level of accountability been more significant than in the critical care environment, where patients are highly complex and vulnerable to the risks associated with hospitalization. Indeed, technological advancements and evidence-based practices in ICUs, where the majority of critical care patients can be found, have begun to focus quality and safety measures as much on preventing harm as on restoring health.

Publication of the Institute of Medicine[1,2] reports and dissemination of their findings related to medical errors and complications has produced intense media coverage on the issue of safety in our health care systems. The result has been increased consumer demands for health care organizations to measure their performance and report their outcomes. Most recently, this heightened scrutiny has led payers to outline plans to deny reimbursement for specific hospital-acquired health conditions.[3] There has been an unprecedented level of action from organizations, professional associations, regulators, accrediting bodies, and consumer groups to make significant changes to their respective agendas to achieve better safety effectiveness, patient centeredness, timeliness, efficiency, and equity.[4]

One example of an action to address the Institute of Medicine concerns was taken in 2003 by the American Association of Critical Care Nurses (AACN), the largest nursing specialty organization in the world. In response to the growing pressures on quality and safety, a growing nursing shortage, and workplace issues, the AACN called upon critical care nurses to assemble for a greater national purpose. One result of this call to action was the Beacon Award for Critical Care Excellence. The Beacon Award recognizes individual critical care units that meet high quality standards, providing exceptional care of patients and patients' families while fostering and sustaining healthy work environments.[5] Recognizing excellence, defined simply as "superior quality," is the primary objective of the Beacon Award. This article introduces the AACN Beacon Award as a framework for quality and discusses the Beacon Award journey.

[a] Adult Critical Care Services and the Neurosciences, Clarian Health Partners, Room A5237, Clarian Health, Methodist Hospital, I-65 at 21st Street, Indianapolis, IN 46206-1367, USA
[b] American Association of Critical Care Nurses Certification Corporation, Aliso Viejo, CA, USA
* Adult Critical Care Services and the Neurosciences, Clarian Health Partners, Room A5237, Clarian Health, Methodist Hospital, I-65 at 21st Street, Indianapolis, IN 46206-1367.
E-mail address: kdreed@clarian.org

Crit Care Nurs Clin N Am 20 (2008) 383–391
doi:10.1016/j.ccell.2008.08.002

ccnursing.theclinics.com

More than 5 million patients are admitted annually to one or more of 6000 critical care units in the United States.[6] Since 1991, treatment for more acute, life-threatening conditions such as hemodynamic abnormalities, multiple system organ failure, sepsis, and shock has continued to rise.[6] Many experts suggest that multiple factors are contributing to this increase, including the ability to more effectively treat these types of patients and the aging of the population in the United States. Whatever the cause, these demographics illustrate the imperative that has prompted the AACN to action. Starting with the crucial question of what a unit that provides excellent patient care would look like, the team charged with developing the process and criteria for the award was given four goals to pursue: (1) to recognize excellence in critical care environments; (2) to recognize excellence of quality measures, processes, structures, and outcomes; (3) to recognize excellence in collaboration, communication, and partnerships that support a healing and humane environment; and (4) to develop a program that contributes to AACN's mission, vision, and values.[7]

From the four goals listed, six categories of evaluation were identified: (1) innovation/recruitment and retention, (2) education/training/mentoring, (3) evidence-based practice/research, (4) patient outcomes, (5) the healing environment, and (6) leadership/organizational ethics. The categories were selected to provide a comprehensive picture of a given critical care unit's culture. They were intended to be inclusive of a myriad of factors that have been associated with superior quality and excellence, including communication and collaboration among caregivers, involvement of the family in the patient's care, and autonomy in professional nursing practice.

Each of the six categories includes a series of Beacon Award application questions that were developed to focus on the unit's structure, processes, and outcomes from a multidisciplinary perspective.[7] The composite picture of the answers to the questions represents forty-two criteria that provide a synthesis of quantitative and qualitative data related to quality. Predetermined standards for each of the criteria were derived from national benchmarks, research, regulatory standards, and expert multidisciplinary consensus. Sources, including several citations from management/leadership based literature, are cited as evidence to support the criteria.

THE BEACON AWARD CRITERIA

Used as a framework for quality and safety, the Beacon Award criteria align in many ways with the Donabedian Model of Patient Safety,[8] which has long served as a unifying framework for examining health services and assessing patient outcomes.[9] The model developed by Avedis Donabedian[8] identifies practitioner performance, which consists of technical competence and interpersonal skills, as making up the core of quality.[10] Technical competence refers to the skills, knowledge, and judgment needed to identify and implement the most effective care strategies. The measurement of technical competence is consistent with best practice and is considered in terms of the future state desired. Maintaining interpersonal relationships, including teamwork and communication, is often ignored yet is a vitally important part of the core of quality and can have a dramatic impact on patient outcomes.[10] Only recently, many authorities have begun to assert the importance of interpersonal relationships in health care[11-13] and to identify these relationships as the key to halting the epidemic of treatment-related harm to patients and the continued erosion of the bottom line in health care organizations.[11]

Several Beacon Award criteria assess technical competence and interpersonal relationships. By including both of these elements of practitioner performance in the criteria, the AACN has established a mechanism to measure the core of quality and allow for the comprehensive evaluation of information from which inferences can be drawn related to excellence.

When assessing the quality of care, the Donabedian Model identifies three elements of care to evaluate quality. Specifically, it identifies (1) structure (ie, how care is organized) plus (2) process (ie, what is done by caregivers), which influences (3) outcomes (ie, the health care results achieved).[14] Others have later added the context, or culture, in which care is delivered to the model.[15] This three-part approach to quality assessment is possible only because good structure increases the likelihood of good process, and good process increases the likelihood of good outcome.[10]

Structure is defined as how care is organized and is often left out of quality measurement, despite growing evidence of its importance in optimizing patient outcomes. It includes a variety of variables that help to establish the foundation for processes to be most effective, including leadership structure, staff orientation and ongoing competency, communication and collaboration among caregivers, and staffing. Process measures include the interventions that we provide that help to reduce the risk of an adverse outcome. They are usually expressed as rates, such as what percentage of patients on ventilators have their head of bed elevated to at least 30 degrees to prevent ventilator-associated pneumonia. Outcome measures include clearly defined numerators and denominators and describe the results achieved. For example, the total number of catheter-related bloodstream infections per 1000 catheter days, considered an avoidable complication, is an outcome measure that is frequently reported in critical care units.

THE BEACON JOURNEY

Depending on the current environment of an individual critical care unit and the extent to which all three dimensions (structure, process, outcomes) of the Donabedian Model are in place, pursuing the Beacon Award can be a challenging journey. The initial step in the journey should be to conduct an assessment of the current state of readiness. An audit tool (**Table 1**) is provided on the AACN Web site at http://www.aacn.org/AACN/ICURecog.nsf/vwdoc/MainPage to assist units in identifying their current performance relative to the standards. The audit tool will help to identify the magnitude of the changes that will be needed to be successful in creating an environment that aligns with the Beacon Award criteria. In addition to the Beacon Award criteria, the audit tool identifies the standards for each criterion and enables work to be prioritized based on whether the unit is on target, working on meeting, or needs to start work on meeting the standard. The tool also identifies the six categories previously mentioned and the criteria associated with each of the categories.

In some cases, the Beacon Award journey will require a unit-based transformational change. As with all cultural change, time, patience, and persistence are needed to reach a desired future. The most general lesson to be learned from the most successful change efforts is that the change process goes through a series of phases that, in total, usually requires a considerable length of time. Skipping steps creates only an illusion of speed and never produces a satisfying result.[16]

Creating an effective quality and safety program requires that structures are in place to support processes and outcomes. Leadership is an essential component of any structure[14] and will provide the foundation for other structural components of quality. An effective leadership structure enables effective communication, incorporates diverse expertise, and provides the resources and support necessary to produce transformational change. When pursuing the Beacon Award, the formation of a group of leaders that are also key stakeholders in the process is vitally important to the effort. The goal is to identify three to five key individuals who can lead the way by bringing others on board with any changes that will be needed. It is important to include respected and influential formal and informal leaders in this group. Formal leaders are needed to support changes and persuade other leaders of the direction to be taken. Informal leaders generally have a better sense of what is happening and what is needed to implement effective changes. This initial group should be powerful in terms of the positions they hold in the organization, the reputations they have, the skills they bring, the strength of their relationships, and the influence they can exert.[16]

Leaders will also set the vision for the work to be done. This is a crucial step in successful transformational change as it serves to unite others toward a common goal. Without a sensible vision, a transformation effort can easily dissolve into a list of confusing and incompatible projects that can take the group in the wrong direction.[16] Once a vision is established and communicated, it can inspire people to action. In general, people will not be willing to change unless there is a useful purpose for doing so. The vision must be compelling enough to move all three components of the Donabedian trilogy and establish a connection between structure, process, and outcome. A rich array of structural measures are associated with patient safety,[16] and many of them have a dramatic effect on the ability to improve processes and outcomes. Implementing effective multidisciplinary rounding is one example of a structural change that has been identified to decrease the length of stay, the rate of ventilator-associated pneumonia, and the rate of catheter-related bloodstream infection and improve overall mortality rates.[17] The task of multidisciplinary rounding must be initiated in such away that it is connected to the overall vision. When multidisciplinary rounding is aligned with the vision, people will see the value of the work and participate with enthusiasm.

A compelling vision must also be communicated and embraced. In the most successful transformation efforts, leaders use all existing communication channels to broadcast the vision.[16] They energize ritualistic methods of communication, including committee meetings, E-mails, newsletters, and postings, and turn them into dynamic dialog that inspires others in discussion about exciting change. By this important step, large numbers of people will be engaged to identify and implement effective quality processes. Because process measures are linked to what caregivers do to influence outcomes, it becomes vital that caregivers be involved early in this step on the Beacon journey. For example, unit-based practice councils can actively review research findings and

Table 1
Beacon Award adult ICU categories and questions audit tool "Are you ready for Beacon?"

Recruitment/Retention	Standard	We Need to StartThis	We are Working onThis	We are on Target or Better
How frequently do you conduct unit specific satisfaction surveys (includes physicians, nurses, and allied health professionals)?	Every 2 years			
How frequently are unit-based meetings conducted for unit-based education and/or information sharing/dialog?	Two times per month			
What is the number of all nursing staff that have been employed in your unit for greater than 5 years?	>50%			
Do you have a recognition program or an incentive program that acknowledges employees on your unit for length of service?	Yes			
How many times per day does nursing leadership (director, manager, manager proxy like charge nurse, assistant manager, house supervisors) make rounds on the unit?	Three times per day			
What is the number of nursing personnel (RNs, LPNs, UAPs, Unit Secretary) FTEs/direct report ratio on your unit?	15 to 1			
Of the last 10 new hires, how many were recruited by your existing staff?	10 out of 10			

Education/Training/Mentoring	Standard	We Need to StartThis	We are Working onThis	We are on Target or Better
How frequently is continuing education provided on the unit specific to the needs of the staff, organization, and/or population?	5 Hours per month			
What is the number of CCRNs/CCNSs in relationship to total number of RN staff in your unit?	65%			
Is there an incentive to become CCRN or CCNS certified?	Yes			
Upon completion of orientation, does the new hire evaluate their orientation process, including needs assessment, customization of orientation to learning needs/experience level, and preceptor experience?	Yes			

	Standard	We Need to Start This	We are Working on This	We are on Target or Better
Do your yearly competency validation requirements meet the criteria of high risk/low volume procedures, patient safety, skills assessment, and quality indicators based on scope of care/service, medical error reports, and regulatory updates?	Yes			
Is there a formal mentoring between novice nurses and expert nurses after orientation?	Yes			
Does your unit use the AACN Standards for Acute and Critical Care Nursing to evaluate professional nursing practice?	Yes			
Evidence-Based Practice/Research	**Standard**	**We Need to Start This**	**We are Working on This**	**We are on Target or Better**
Are your unit policies and procedures based on nationally recognized levels of evidence/best practice?	Yes			
How frequently is routine surveillance of the research and literature done to support practice review and change?	One time per month			
Do you have nurses based on your unit who are participating in clinical research?	Yes			
Patient Outcomes	**Standard**	**We need to Start This**	**We are Working on This**	**We are on Target or Better**
What is your unit rate of unplanned extubations per 1000 ventilator days?	<3%			
What is your unit-based rate of catheter-associated urinary tract infections per 1000 device days?	<5.6/1000			
What is your unit-based rate of central line-related bloodstream infections per 1000 device days?	<1.6/1000			
What is your unit-based rate of ventilator-associated pneumonia per 1000 ventilator days?	<5.8/1000			
What is your unit-based rate of pressure ulcers or greater than or equal to grade II per 1000 patient days (excluding pressure ulcers evident on admission to the ICU)?	<3.7/1000			
What is your unit-based rate of deep vein thrombosis per 1000 patient days?	<13%			
What is the medication error rate in your unit per 1000 doses?	No standard			

(continued on next page)

Table 1
(continued)

Recruitment/Retention	Standard	We Need to Start This	We are Working on This	We are on Target or Better
Healing Environment	**Standard**	**We Need to Start This**	**We are Working on This**	**We are on Target or Better**
How frequently does an interdisciplinary team make bedside rounds to influence/change/augment the plan of care?	One time per week			
Can the nurses in your unit, based on patient assessment, initiate requests for interdisciplinary referrals of services?	Yes			
Are nursing assignments made based on patient acuity and competencies of the nurses?	Yes			
Are changes in the plan of care made based on patient condition and review of interdisciplinary documentation?	Yes			
Does the patient room have visual access to the outside (the hospital) environment?	Yes			
What is the number of AACN Bold Voices Commitment statements signed RN staff in your unit? (If your unit has not seen the Bold Voices Commitment site, go to https://my.aacn.org/ecomtpro/timssnet/actboldly/aacn_actboldly_frontpage.cfm.)	100%			
When the goals of care change from acute to comfort care for the patient, do you initiate palliative, end-of-life, and/or hospice care in the ICU?	Yes			
Do you have a unit policy in place to describe patient and family involvement in open or negotiated visiting hours and the family presence during procedures and/or cardiopulmonary resuscitation?	Yes			
Do you have a specific method of assessing and documenting pain in the nonresponsive patient?	Yes			
Is there a mechanism to debrief unit-based nursing staff after stressful incidences, including end-of-life, interpersonal, and abusive/violent situations?	Yes			

	Standard	We Need to Start This	We are Working on This	We are on Target or Better
Based on assessed patient needs, do the nurses have access to cultural and spiritual resources appropriate to the patient population?	Yes			
How many times a day is there collaborative communication to determine patient care goals and to develop/change the patient plan of care?	At least one per day			
Leadership/Organizational Ethics				
What percentage of the unit nursing leadership was selected from the staff in the unit (eg, nurse manager, assistant manager, charge nurses, APNs)? (Staff selected for leadership first number/total leadership second number)	>75%			
How many of all RN staff on the unit (all roles) belong to a professional nursing organization? (RN staff in professional organization first number/total RN staff second number)	75%			
Do the standards of the unit leadership team include joint leadership accountability between the nurse manager/director and the medical director?	Yes			
Do nurses and physicians in your unit participate in open dialog and education during daily interdisciplinary rounds?	Yes			
Does every member of the unit staff have accountability for identifying issues requiring process improvement?	Yes			
What is the ratio between patient issues and non-patient (staff, physician, organizational) issues in your units' ethics consults for the past year? (Patient issues first number/non-patient issues second number)	No standard			

Abbreviations: FTEs, full-time equivalents; UAPs, unlicensed assistive personnel.
The Beacon Award adult ICU categories and questions audit tool is used with permission from the American Association of Critical Care Nurses. Available at: http://www.aacn.org/AACN/ICURecog.nsf/vwdoc/MainPage.

determine the evidence-based processes that will most likely minimize the adverse outcome of urinary tract infection. Armed with this information, they can be instrumental in influencing the practice of others and empowering them to take action.

When it becomes clear that outcomes improve through process changes, people will see clearly what the Beacon journey is producing and will join the ranks of those that led the way. Systematically planning for and creating short-term wins will improve the momentum of the transformational changes and allow for celebrations along the way.[16] After process changes have been implemented, outcome measures will most likely begin to improve. The Beacon Award criterion includes identified, pre-determined outcome measures based on nationally recognized standards for identifying the numerator and denominator to normalize raw numbers. This analysis allows for the reporting and benchmarking of performance through meaningful data. To create short-term wins, data need to be shared in ways that convey information with a quick glance. Creating line graphs, bar graphs, or pie charts is useful for this purpose.

Lastly, transformational change involves institutionalizing change and making it a part of the culture. Two factors become important in this step. The first is a conscious attempt to show people how the new approaches have helped to improve performance. Once again, this requires communication to help people make the connection. The second and most important factor is ensuring that the next generation of leaders carries the same message and that they become champions of the change effort. In this way, the change is passed on and eventually becomes "the way we do things."

THE BEACON AWARD APPLICATION

The Beacon Award application includes 42 scored questions and requires both quantitative and qualitative responses. The quantitative responses are of three types: yes or no, ratio, or numerator/denominator. Additionally, it is expected that each of the responses are supported with qualitative documentation, limited to 300 words and consistent with the quantitative responses. The qualitative portion of the application provides the unit with the opportunity to highlight performance improvement strategies, innovation, evidence-based practice, the overall health of the work environment, and additional structure, process, or outcome data. It is not necessary to include graphs or charts in the narrative response; however, each unit should be prepared to produce this information if audited through an established random selection process.

The responses to each of the questions should demonstrate a multidisciplinary effort in the pursuit of excellence. This demonstration will strengthen the application by illustrating the effectiveness of interpersonal relationships in driving quality efforts. It is also desirable that leaders and staff participate in writing narrative responses and in reviewing the application before submission. This joint participation will help to demonstrate that a vision for quality has permeated the culture and includes a staff-driven commitment to excellence.

Nonmembers of the AACN can apply for the Beacon Award for Critical Care Excellence. Each critical care unit must apply individually for the award by accessing the online application process at http://www.aacn.org/AACN/ICURecog. nsf/vwdoc/MainPage. Once the application has been initiated, it can be saved so questions can be amended up to the time the application is submitted. After it is submitted, the application is considered final, and no further changes can be made. There is no deadline for submission of the application.

A panel of experts has been selected by AACN to review the Beacon Award application. The panel is made up of individuals who are chosen based on their knowledge and understanding of the critical care environment and their demonstrated commitment to supporting excellence in critical care. Each application is reviewed blindly by a minimum of three expert panel members. Quantitative review includes identification of whether the unit meets, exceeds, or does not meet the standards outlined for the criteria. Qualitative review of the application gives the reviewer additional information to provide a final determination of their recommendation for award status.

Applications for the Beacon Award are reviewed by the expert panel on a quarterly basis. In many cases, the panel will request additional information before making a decision about the award status. If this occurs, the applying unit is given a maximum of 60 days to submit further documentation to strengthen the application before its final review. When the award is bestowed upon a unit, it is considered active for 1 year from the month of receipt of the award. A critical care unit can apply for the award every year.

Beacon Award winners are publicly recognized by AACN at the local and national level through press releases and their internal publication, AACN News, which is distributed to 90,000 nurses across the country and abroad. Hospitals have marketed receipt of the award in various ways, including interstate billboards, Web site announcements, and recruitment events. As of May 1, 2008, 120 critical care units have been recognized with the Beacon Award. Seventeen of these 120 units have received the award twice and one unit three times. A complete listing of the awarded units is available on the AACN Beacon Award Web site.

SUMMARY

A new paradigm for quality and safety in health care has placed increasing pressure on providers to improve their delivery systems and document their outcomes. This challenge is particularly true for critical care units where patients have complex needs and are at the greatest risk for complications. For critical care units to be successful, the multidisciplinary team must embrace a model for quality and safety that enables assessment and monitoring of improvement activities.

The Beacon Award for Critical Care Excellence provides a solid framework for assessing, measuring, and documenting quality. It can guide a critical care unit on a transformational journey that will include development of structures, processes, and outcomes that are supported by practitioner performance, including technical competence and intrapersonal skills. Each of these elements of quality must be developed and fine-tuned to establish a foundation that fosters a culture of excellence and allows it to grow and flourish.

ACKNOWLEDGMENTS

The author wishes to acknowledge Justine Medina, the Director of Professional Practice and Programs at the American Association of Critical Care Nurses, for her contribution in the preparation of this article.

REFERENCES

1. Corrigan J, Kohn L, Donaldson MS, editors. To err is human: building a safer health system. Washington, DC: National Academy Press; 1999. p. 1–6.
2. Institute of Medicine. Crossing the quality chasm: a new healthcare system for the 21st century. Washington (DC): National Academy Press; 2001.
3. Pear R. Medicare says it will not cover hospital errors. New York Times. August 19, 2007. Available at: http://www.nytimes.com. Accessed April 12, 2008.
4. Committee on Redesigning Health Insurance Performance Measures, Payment, and Performance Improvement Programs. Performance measurement: accelerating improvement. Series: pathways to quality health care. Institute of Medicine. Washington, DC: National Academy Press; 2006. Available at: http://www.nap.edu/catalog/11517.html. Accessed April 28, 2008.
5. Ulrich T, Woods D, Hart KA, et al. Critical care nurses' work environments value of excellence in Beacon units and magnet organizations. Crit Care Nurse 2007;27(3):68–77.
6. Society of Critical Care Medicine. Critical care statistics in the United States 2006. Available at: http://www.sccm.org./AboutSCCM/Public%20Relations/Pages/Statistics. Accessed April 10, 2008.
7. American Association of Critical Care Nurses. Beacon award for critical care excellence 2003. Available at: http://www.aacn.org/AACN/ICURecog.nsf/vwdoc/MainPage. Accessed April 4, 2008.
8. Donabedian A. The definition of quality and approaches to its assessment. Ann Arbor (MI): Health Administration Press; 1980.
9. Baker DP, Gustafson S, Beaubien J, et al. Medical teamwork and patient safety: the evidence-based relation [literature review]. AHRQ Publication No. 05–0053. Rockville (MD): Agency for Healthcare Research and Quality; 2005. Available at: http://www.ahrq.gov/qual/medteam. Accessed May 2, 2008.
10. Donabedian A. The quality of care. JAMA 1988; 260(12):1743–8.
11. American Association of Critical Care Nurses. AACN standards for establishing and sustaining healthy work environments: a journey to excellence. Aliso Viejo (CA): American Association of Critical Care Nurses; 2005.
12. Rutherford P, Lee B, Greier A. Transforming care at the bedside. IHI Innovation Series white paper. Boston: Institute for Healthcare Improvement; 2004.
13. Joint Commission. Reducing medical errors: a review of innovative strategies to improve patient safety. Testimony of Dennis S. O'Leary. Washington, DC, May 8, 2002. Available at: http://www.jointcommission.org/NewsRoom/OnCapitolHill/. Accessed May 4, 2008.
14. Pronovost P, Miller M, Wachter RM. Tracking progress in patient safety: an elusive target. JAMA 2006;296(6):696–9.
15. Pronovost P, Holzmueller CG, Nedham DM, et al. How will we know patients are safer? An organization-wide approach to measuring and improving safety. Crit Care Med 2006;34(7):1988–95.
16. Kotter JP. Leading change: why transformational efforts fail. Harvard Business Review. March–April, 1995;59–67.
17. Institute for Healthcare Improvement. Improvement report. Multidisciplinary rounds: not more work but the work. Available at: http://www.inhi.org/topics/improvement/improvementmethods/improvementstories/multiddiscipinaryrounds. Accessed May 2, 2008.

The American Association of Critical Care Nurses Standards for Establishing and Sustaining Healthy Work Environments: Off the Printed Page and into Practice

John F. Dixon, MSN, RN, NE-BC

KEYWORDS

- Healthy work environment • Standards
- Acute and critical care
- Evidence-based nursing practice

In January 2005, the American Association of Critical-Care Nurses (AACN) led out and, using a bold voice, released the *AACN Standards for Establishing and Sustaining Healthy Work Environments: A Journey to Excellence*.[1] This publication was the culmination of work from an expert panel combined with the input of 50 additional reviewers representing various roles from across the nation. The impetus for this initiative was the growing body of evidence that unhealthy work environments have an adverse impact not only on patients and families but on employees and organizations as well. As a result, the AACN made a commitment in 2001 to make healthy work environments (HWEs) one of the association's key and ongoing initiatives.[1] The publication's debut at a Washington, DC press conference included AACN representatives and key health care stake holders, such as Dennis S. O'Leary, MD, then Joint Commission President. Initial feedback from AACN members through its board advisory teams indicated that of the six standards, skilled communication was a pressing priority. This view reinforced the findings from the Silence Kills study, a cosponsored project by the AACN and VitalSmarts.[2] Since its release, others have used their bold voices in support of the standards as collaborative partners or through endorsements from professional organizations, research, and publications in addition to educational programming, such as that produced through the Joint Commission Resources.[3–7]

The six standards are skilled communication, true collaboration, effective decision making, appropriate staffing, meaningful recognition, and authentic leadership. Each standard begins with a call to action focusing on a primary imperative. Next is a condensed review of pertinent literature for that particular standard, with references and additional suggested readings listed at the end of the chapter. The guidelines that follow are listed as critical elements and define not only individual responsibilities but those of organizations as well. By including both aspects, we are reminded that an initiative of this magnitude can begin with one person but truly requires a collective and

The Center for Nursing Education and Research, Baylor University Medical Center, 3500 Gaston Avenue, Dallas, TX 75246, USA
E-mail address: johndi@baylorhealth.edu

Crit Care Nurs Clin N Am 20 (2008) 393–401
doi:10.1016/j.ccell.2008.08.010

unified effort at all levels. Of note, the critical elements are written in active rather than passive voice, emphasizing the action-oriented approach needed to establish and sustain such work environments. So, with a copy in hand and your outcome goal defined, you may find yourself asking "How and where do I start?" and "Can I be the one to initiate this journey to excellence?" The answer is a definite yes. The purpose of this article is to introduce the AACN's standards for establishing and sustaining an HWE and to discuss ways to implement the standards in the acute and critical care workplace.

DEVELOPING A VALUE EQUATION

Professional nursing practice does not take place in a vacuum but rather within some type of environment. These settings are typically organizations, such as hospitals and clinics. The ability of the nurse to practice professional nursing has linkages with the environment in which that practice takes place. Although it may be possible for professional practice to take place in an unhealthy environment, it is not likely to be sustained. Poor communication and collaboration, inadequate information with which to make effective decisions, staffing that does not match the needs of patients, disingenuous recognition, and absence of leadership create multiple obstacles and burdens in the delivery of care. These deficits have an impact on unit function, morale, quality, and public relations, creating a slow downward spiral. Nurses leave such settings to seek environments in which making their optimal contribution is facilitated and supported through healthy structures, processes, and outcomes.

To prepare for introducing the HWE standards, take time to develop a value equation to answer the question, "What's in it for me?" When opening dialog with colleagues, ask if they have ever thought about the amount of time they spend in the work environment. For example, a person working 36 hours per week minus 3 weeks of vacation logs a total of 1764 worked hours across 1 year. With a total of 8760 hours in a year, these worked hours then account for 20.1% of that person's life annually. The question to then ask is "If you are going to spend one fifth of your life each year in the work environment, wouldn't you want that to be an HWE, an environment that you don't mind returning to shift after shift, versus an unhealthy environment?"

"What's in it for me?" is equally important to organizations as well. Nationally, patient outcomes are increasingly evident in the spotlight. Measurements have evolved over the years from individual hospitals measuring self-identified indicators internally to increasing requirements from external agencies and the publication of report cards for the general public.[8-10] Even as far back as the 1980s, work environment aspects, such as collaboration, were shown to have an impact on patient outcomes. Knaus and colleagues[11] found that mortality rates were lower than predicted in intensive care units, in which interaction and coordination between staff and physicians were better. More recently, a Canadian study found lower rates of 30-day mortality in hospitals with higher nurse-physician collaboration scores.[12]

Facilities with HWEs may experience operational and financial benefits, such as increased patient volumes from steerage of patients by payers; reduced care delivery costs increasing operating margins; and other benefits, such as better bond ratings and enhanced patient satisfaction and reputation as a result of high-quality patient outcomes. Internally, such facilities may experience greater stability and better cost management through fewer staff sick days, recruitment of higher caliber applicants for open positions, less staff turnover, higher staff satisfaction and morale, consistently higher personnel performance ratings, and achievement of institutional goals. Such effects are definitely key strategic initiatives for facilities and will make even a stronger argument for actively investing in and supporting structures and processes that create and sustain HWEs if future research supports such associations.

CREATING AWARENESS

So where do you start? Perhaps you think the six standards are just what your work environment needs, and you want to implement all these right away. Although such enthusiasm and energy are commendable, realistically trying to implement everything at once may lead to failure. The scope of such a task can far exceed available resources, people, and energy, resulting in disappointing outcomes and a draining of the initial drive. To avoid such a situation, start with an introduction of the standards to individuals and groups, formally and informally. From these interactions, you should get a sense of whether they see relevance in the standards related to their current work situation, feel a need for making a change, and are willing to be part of the journey.

If your organization provides e-mail accounts, consider sending an e-mail to key individuals you know with a brief introduction to the standards, along with the Web link to the AACN's HWE Web page.[13] The advantage of providing the Web address is twofold. First, this Web page includes downloadable copies of the executive summary or a complete version of the HWE standards. Although you could have attached these files to the e-mail you sent, by not doing so, you avoid the risk for causing the receiver's e-mail to exceed its allotted memory. When exceeded, e-mail typically locks up and is not functional again until large files, such as these, are deleted. Thus, your e-mail risks deletion without being read. Also some organizations have policy restrictions on the use of attached files. Those who are constantly in jeopardy of hitting that maximum memory limit appreciate this courteous consideration. Second, the Web page itself is a rich resource of additional information related to the HWE, and thus allows the reader opportunity to explore. If e-mail is not an option, download and print copies of the HWE executive summary from the Web page. You can then send these printouts to key individuals by means of interoffice mail, along with a brief introductory note. Be sure to include the Web link in your note. Additional individual contacts can occur during casual conversations by asking colleagues if they have heard about the HWE standards, and, if not, share with them some key points. Solicit their initial reactions to the standards and thoughts about implementing these (eg, do they think it is needed; if so, is it doable and what would be a first priority).

More formal introductions of the standards usually take place in structured forums, such as council, committee, and task force meetings. Request to attend such a meeting to present an HWE overview as part of the agenda. Before the meeting, look at the agenda and try to map any of the topics to one of the six standards. During your presentation, make reference to how a particular agenda item links to one of the standards. Such associations aid in validating the relevance of the standards for the group, making them "real." As with individual contacts, close your presentation by soliciting initial reactions and thoughts. If you are not comfortable making formal presentations to groups, explore the possibility of using a resource from the HWE Speakers Bureau, found on the AACN's HWE Web site. If you are a regular member of a particular group, review the meeting minutes over several months looking for linkages to the six standards. Depending on how long you have been a member of the group and after you have introduced HWE to them, introduce the idea of organizing agenda items according to the six standards. An advantage to using the HWE as a framework is that you can easily identify areas that are not being routinely addressed but probably need to be.

Now that you have started building HWE awareness, the question is what to do next. Think back on what kind of reactions you have encountered. What did individuals and groups see as a first priority of the six standards? Use such cues and clues to guide you. Think back to common themes that consistently come up again and again in the work environment. Although such qualitative data are a rich resource, readily available quantitative data may provide additional insights. Numbers data may be in the form of employee survey results, risk management reports, and quality and outcomes results.

DEVELOPING YOUR ACTION PLAN

Once you and your colleagues have targeted a standard to work on, talk about what is your measurable baseline, or your anchor point. If you do not have a defined starting point for comparison, you cannot know if you are moving forward. Sometimes, baseline data may already be routinely collected, such as some type of ongoing quarterly report. In other instances, you may find that your first step is to collect baseline data yourself. Taking on such a task may sound daunting, but the critical elements for each standard can serve as a guide and a resource for what to assess and measure. For example, if you identified skilled communication as the first standard to work on, a simple questionnaire could be developed using that standard's critical elements (**Tables 1** and **2**).

For this skilled communication assessment, two perspectives of the same critical elements were developed: a self-evaluation and a unit evaluation. Staff members are asked to rate themselves against the critical element statements and then evaluate the unit as a whole. When the data are analyzed, the summary results give a picture of how individuals see themselves versus how they see everyone else. These baseline data may reveal that individuals see themselves as exemplars of skilled communication but not the rest of the unit. This contradiction serves as a learning event in itself, because everyone develops a new awareness of the unit's current mental model. After additional activities and interventions, this same tool could be used again. The postmeasurement results could be compared with the premeasurement results to determine the effectiveness of the unit's efforts to address skilled communication.

Developing a questionnaire does take some time and, typically, does not have established validity and reliability unless rigorous effort is invested, which prolongs your implementation. There may be valid and reliable tools available that you can use for doing your measurements, however. For example, if you are interested in working on the true collaboration standard, you

---

Table 1
Skilled communication questionnaire: self-evaluation

Rating Scale	1 = Rarely, 2 = Occasionally, 3 = Usually, 4 = Consistently	Rate Yourself
	I actively work on improving my communication skills.	
	I seek feedback from others on how my communication style is received.	
	I ask questions and engage in discussion before forming an opinion on an issue.	
	When presented with a conflict situation, I deal with it.	
	I manage conflict situations using a positive assertive manner.	
	When required, I can effectively negotiate.	
	I advocate for patients.	
	I advocate for families.	
	I advocate for staff.	
	I take the time to carefully listen to what others have to say.	
	When presented with a problem, I complain.	
	When presented with a problem, I identify at least two practical/realistic solutions.	
	I work on achieving desirable patient outcomes.	
	I work on achieving desirable unit outcomes.	
	I promote collaborative relationships among colleagues.	
	I invite and hear all relevant perspectives on an issue.	
	I build consensus through goodwill and mutual respect.	
	I work to ensure everyone has a common understanding on an issue.	
	My actions are consistent with my words.	
	I give feedback to others when their actions are not consistent with their words.	
	I engage in abusive or disrespectful behavior in the workplace.	
	When a person acts in an abusive or disrespectful manner, I confront him or her.	
	I communicate effectively and share information with patients.	
	I communicate effectively and share information with visitors.	
	I communicate effectively and share information with the health care team.	
	I access my e-mail.	
	I review the Communication Book.	
	I check my unit mailbox.	
	I keep up with the information posted on the bulletin boards.	
	I take the time to formally evaluate how my communication has an impact on clinical outcomes.	
	I take the time to formally evaluate how my communication has an impact on the work environment.	

Courtesy of J.F. Dixon, MSN, RN, Dallas, TX.

might choose the Jefferson Scale of Attitudes Toward Physician-Nurse Collaboration.[14] When using an established tool, look for other instances in the literature in which it has been used. See if these situations are similar to how you would like to use the tool, and note the processes followed and any lessons learned. Of great importance is to ask the tool's author for permission to use it. Some tools may have user fees associated with them, whereas others do not. The author may request a copy of your raw data so that she or he can add those to an ongoing compilation of results.

Another usual first step in building an HWE is to investigate what is available in the literature. This exploration should give you ideas of how best to chart your course. Another method for establishing a baseline is to identify best practices within your organization. After identifying your priority standard, review the critical elements and look for work units in which it is common to hear comments about excellence related to that standard.

Table 2
Skilled communication questionnaire: unit evaluation

Rating Scale	1 = Rarely, 2 = Occasionally, 3 = Usually, 4 = Consistently	Rate Others in the Unit as a Whole
They actively work on improving their communication skills.		
They seek feedback from others on how their communication style is received.		
They ask questions and engage in discussion before forming an opinion on an issue.		
When presented with a conflict situation, they deal with it.		
They manage conflict situations using a positive assertive manner.		
When required, they can effectively negotiate.		
They advocate for patients.		
They advocate for families.		
They advocate for staff.		
They take the time to carefully listen to what others have to say.		
When presented with a problem, they complain.		
When presented with a problem, they identify at least two practical/realistic solutions.		
They work on achieving desirable patient outcomes.		
They work on achieving desirable unit outcomes.		
They promote collaborative relationships among colleagues.		
They invite and hear all relevant perspectives on an issue.		
They build consensus through goodwill and mutual respect.		
They work to ensure everyone has a common understanding on an issue.		
Their actions are consistent with their words.		
They give feedback to others when others' actions are not consistent with their words.		
They engage in abusive or disrespectful behavior in the workplace.		
When a person acts in an abusive or disrespectful manner, they confront him or her.		
They communicate effectively and share information with patients.		
They communicate effectively and share information with visitors.		
They communicate effectively and share information with the health care team.		
They are current with information found in e-mails, Communication Book, mailboxes, and bulletin boards.		
They take the time to formally evaluate how their communication has an impact on clinical outcomes.		
They take the time to formally evaluate how their communication has an impact on the work environment.		

Courtesy of J.F. Dixon, MSN, RN, Dallas, TX.

Identify what are the best practices in that area, and explore what structures and processes they have in place to support and sustain such exemplar performance. If you discover such a model unit, be careful of the temptation to quickly copy those practices and roll them out house-wide in a "cookie cutter" fashion. That unit's best practices may not be readily transferable or generalizable because of the uniqueness of that unit in comparison to all the others. For other units, foundational work to establish certain structures may be needed before introducing these best practices. In other areas, modifications may be needed to create a best fit and relevance for the target unit and its staff. For still other areas, these best practices may not be applicable at all; an original approach may be needed because of the unit's individuality. Although all units share the same end goal of establishing and sustaining HWEs, the journey to excellence that each takes does not have to be exactly the same.

The critical elements can also be used to perform a gap analysis on your unit—what do you definitely have in place, what is sort of in place, and

Table 3
Examples of linkages between a healthy work environment and operations

Healthy work environment	Annual National Database of Nursing Quality Indicators Nurse Satisfaction Survey
	Bi-Annual Human Resources Employee Satisfaction Survey
	Shared governance councils
	Reflected in job descriptions and performance evaluation expectations
	House-wide employee town hall meetings
Skilled communication	Policies: zero tolerance, chain of command, stop the line
	Structured patient information on hand-offs
	Patient and staff rounding
	Defined communication pathways among shared governance councils
	Publications: nursing news, E-mail alerts
	Unit staff meetings
	Tracking and trending systems for disruptive communication
	Continuing education programs: conflict management, negotiation, active listening, dialog
	E-mail accounts provided by the organization
Collaboration	Continuing education programs focusing on team training
	Simulation laboratory exercises combining clinical and collaboration competence
	Interdisciplinary rounds
	Interdisciplinary practice council
	Decision authority of shared governance councils
	Continuing education programs: diversity training
Effective decision making	Clearly defined, coordinated, and communicated nursing values and goals from system to unit level
	Data transparency
	Available consults/resources (eg, ethics consult, palliative care team, pain management, clinical nurse specialists, wound and skin care team, clinical dietitians)
	Evidence-based practice initiatives and changes
	Outcomes tracking as a means to evaluate decisions made
Appropriate staffing	Staffing plan for nursing with periodic review and evaluation
	Professional nursing practice model that endorses assignments wherein patient needs are matched to nurse competencies
	Staffing and scheduling systems and policies
	Support services and equipment to enhance safety and efficiency in care delivery (eg, unit-based nurse case manager, patient lift equipment, medication bar coding, on-line documentation, reference systems)
Meaningful recognition	Annual performance appraisals
	Clinical ladders/professional advancement programs
	Excellence in customer service recognition program
	Formal system, hospital, and unit-based recognition programs that encompass a variety of methods
	Annual Nurses' Week celebration
	Annual nursing report (eg, outcomes, posters, presentations, publications, awards)
	Defined plan to submit eligible staff members and units for local and national awards (eg, AACN Circle of Excellence Awards, Beacon Award for Critical Care Excellence)
	Recognition of nursing accomplishments on internal and external Web sites
	Expectation that recognition is not just top down but multidirectional, interdisciplinary, and interdepartmental—everyone's responsibility
	Culture celebrates not only the major accomplishments but daily contributions

(continued on next page)

Table 3 (continued)	
Authentic leadership	One manager to one unit
	Administrative rounding
	Open door communication
	Administration/management initiatives that promote and sustain an HWE
	Nurse leaders have key decision-making roles in all levels of the organizational chart
	Continuing education programs: ongoing leadership development opportunities

what is definitely missing? Have each member of your HWE team do this assessment individually, and then compare your results. This approach allows the team to see where there is definite consensus and variation. For items for which your assessments vary, initiate a dialog about why this may be. From this discussion, you may find that the variation may be caused by other unit variables. For example, something may be seen as definitely present on night shift but definitely missing on day shift; thus, the shift is influencing that particular element. During this discussion, identify if there are contributing factors to be considered, positive and negative. For those items that can facilitate your efforts, discuss how you can make the most of them, and for those items that can hinder your efforts, plan how you can minimize or eliminate these obstacles. During your planning sessions, also consider if there are internal and external resources that you may need or would be helpful and how to tap into those. Such supports may take the form of supplies, communication networks, or specific individuals who can serve as key opinion leaders. Using all data you have collected and discussed, have the team decide which items are of the highest priority and, if addressed, would have the greatest impact on the unit as a whole. Addressing issues that are affecting everyone provides a foundation for dealing with unique issues (eg, shift specific) or might even have a ripple effect and resolve the issue.

Education is a frequently selected initial intervention. Keep in mind that multiple educational initiatives, such as new equipment, revised policies, new order sets, or procedure changes, are common in a dynamic work setting. To prevent direct competition with these initiatives, try to determine which projects are slated for implementation, what are the start dates, and what is the anticipated rollout duration. Although it is impossible to avoid every initiative, knowledge such as this should allow you to make an effective decision regarding timing of your HWE rollout. Remember that not everyone learns in the same manner, so develop your content with several learning methodologies that

engage the learner, consider generational variation, and add a dash of fun. Also listen to current comments from staff about recent projects. If you hear that they are inundated and tired of self-learning modules, avoid using that method. Education often needs supplementation with practice, encouragement, and mentoring. Develop follow-up mechanisms to assist your staff in fully translating their new knowledge into daily practice.

To wrap up your action plan, establish a time line. Having specific dates by which to complete certain interventions keeps everyone moving forward. Without such direction, you risk losing momentum and your well-designed plans slowly fall apart. Dates also create a sense of expectation and accountability. Decide what is going to be your first major end point, how you are going to know you have arrived, and what is going to be your measure. It is possible that this could be several months into the future, and waiting for the major end point could seem to be so distant that individuals may feel a bit discouraged. As a result, build in to your plan some milestones along the journey to your major end point. Communicate accomplishment of these to the team, and celebrate these as evidence of continued progress toward your end goal.

Moving to an HWE can be a big undertaking. You may find your planned interventions did not work out as well as you had hoped. Such backslides should not be seen as failures but as a bump in the road on your journey. You can get over a bump with some extra efforts. This finding is a reality when implementing any plan, because we can only think of possibilities that we can envision, and, obviously, there are more that we have not thought about. Your team may have to regroup periodically and revise some approaches because they are not working as hoped or in response to organizational changes, such as a merger between two units. Keep in mind that an HWE is not static but dynamic. As such, the team needs to be resilient and responsive to such changes so that you can continue to progress forward.

SUSTAINING THE CHANGE

Making a change is a single step; sustaining the change is the journey. Although individual projects are important and contribute to the overall sum of the parts, the HWE needs to be infused into all aspects of operations such that it is an operational norm and not something added on. Threading the standards throughout all aspects of operations ensures that the whole environment is committed rather than just a few stand-alone silos. It may be possible for a single unit to maintain an HWE while surrounded by non-HWE units, but the reality is that these sustaining old patterns create ongoing risk for returning to a prior level of functioning.

Threading begins with recruitment of staff for open positions. Marketing materials should highlight the organization's commitment to an HWE. During the interview process with prospective new hires, behaviorally based interview questions should explore the standards. For example, instead of asking "Do you believe that communication skills are important," ask "Tell me about a time when your communications skills were more important than your clinical skills." Job descriptions and performance evaluations should reflect the organization's commitment to an HWE.

During orientation, aspects of an HWE should be an integral part of the curriculum. The administrative welcome should include a testament to the value and importance that the organization places on an HWE and how the organization holds each employee accountable and responsible for these standards. New hires should expect that the facility can easily articulate what structures and processes they have in place to support and sustain an HWE (**Table 3**). During an internship, if a clinical case is being analyzed, include not only the clinical analysis but how that information would be skillfully communicated, with whom the new hire would need to collaborate, and what information is needed for effective decision making. Aspects of an HWE should integrate somehow with the professional nursing practice model because practice is taking place within that setting. Unit councils should come to consensus on behavioral norms and codes of conduct for their units that are consistent with an HWE, along with a commitment of each member to be accountable for these and to hold their peers accountable as well. Continuing education offerings should reinforce an HWE by integrating it into clinical content or having dedicated programs on topics, such as communication or collaboration. Although verbal testimony to supporting an HWE is a commitment, the evidence is in whether that translates into action— "walking the talk."

SUMMARY

Although you may wish for a rapid overnight change, the reality is that moving to an HWE takes time. An HWE is not a one-time checklist event, over and done. Rather, it is an ongoing and evolving process requiring continued vigilance. Hopefully, you can move beyond individuals participating simply out of compliance and progress to true commitment. Compliance typically takes place only when someone is closely watching. Commitment arises from shared beliefs and values about how the environment needs to be and the willingness to invest the time, resources, and efforts to achieve this goal. By ensuring that key stake holders are involved in all phases of planning, implementing, and evaluating, you can increase the probability for commitment as opposed to compliance. Consistent with the standards, skilled communicators "protect and advance collaborative relationships…invite and hear all relevant perspectives…call upon good will and mutual respect to build consensus and arrive at common understanding."[1] Thus, as you work to put into practice the HWE standards, you must incorporate and practice the expectations as part of the process for developing your plan. You may find that once the HWE initiative has begun, the positive momentum it generates may make the whole process self-renewing. In publishing the HWE standards, the AACN led out, using a bold voice; it is now up to you to move these off the printed page and into practice.

REFERENCES

1. American Association of Critical-Care Nurses. AACN standards for establishing and sustaining healthy work environments: a journey to excellence. Available at: http://www.aacn.org/WD/HWE/Content/hwe-home.pcms?menu=Community. Accessed May 31, 2008.
2. Maxfield D, Grenny J, McMillan R, et al. Silence kills: the seven crucial conversations for healthcare. Provo (UT): VitalSmarts, LC; 2005.
3. American Association of Critical-Care Nurses. Healthy work environments: collaborative partners and endorsements. Available at: http://www.aacn.org/WD/HWE/Content/partners.pcms?menu=Practice. Accessed May 31, 2008.
4. Schmalenberg C, Kramer M. Types of intensive care units with the healthiest, most productive work environments. Am J Crit Care 2007;16(5):458–68.
5. Joint Commission Resources. JCR/AACN 2008 Web-conference Series for Nurses. Available at: http://store.jcrinc.com/JCRStore/FillCatalogAnonymousAction.

do?nocache=jq6HbmKYxR5KXpc7AGSiPRK. Accessed May 31, 2008.

6. Ulrich BT, Lavandero R, Hart KA, et al. Healthy work environments. Critical care nurses' work environments: a baseline status report. Crit Care Nurse 2006;26(5):46–8, 49–50, 52–7.

7. Ulrich BT, Woods D, Hart KA, et al. Critical care nurses' work environments value of excellence in beacon units and magnet organizations. Crit Care Nurse 2007;27(3):68–77.

8. Centers for Medicare and Medicaid Services Hospital Center. Available at: http://www.cms.hhs.gov/center/hospital.asp. Accessed May 31, 2008.

9. National Quality Forum (2004). National Voluntary Consensus Standards for Nursing-Sensitive Care: an initial performance measure set. Available at: http://www.qualityforum.org/publications/reports/nsc.asp. Accessed May 31, 2008.

10. United States Department of Health and Human Services. Hospital compare. Available at: http://www.hospitalcompare.hhs.gov/Hospital/Search/Welcome.asp?version=default&browser=IE%7C6%7CWinXP&language=English&defaultstatus=0&pagelist=Home; 2008. Accessed May 31, 2008.

11. Knaus WA, Draper EA, Wagner DP, et al. An evaluation of outcome from intensive care in major medical centers. Ann Intern Med 1986;104(3):410–8.

12. Estabrooks CA, Midodzi WK, Cummings GG, et al. The impact of hospital nursing characteristics on 30-day mortality. Nurse Res 2005;54(2):74–84.

13. Available at: http://www.aacn.org/WD/HWE/Content/hwehome.pcms?menu=Community. Accessed May 31, 2008.

14. Hojat M. Physician-nurse collaboration. Available at: http://www.jefferson.edu/jmc/crmehc/health/pcollaboration.cfm; 2008. Accessed May 31, 2008.

Integrating Human Caring Science into a Professional Nursing Practice Model

Karen Neil Drenkard, PhD, RN, NEA-BC*

KEYWORDS

- Professional nursing practice model • Human caring
- Decreasing work intensity • Model of care

Current supply and demand projections for registered nurses (RNs) in the United States paint a picture with many gaps. Efforts have been directed to increasing the supply of nurses through increasing enrollments and increasing the number of new graduate nurses. Challenges, such as faculty shortages, exacerbate the problem, hampering the hard work that has been directed at increasing the number of students so that the subsequent supply of nurses is increased. The other half of the equation is improving the retention rate of nurses, especially in hospitals across the country. The nurse leader is required to pay attention to the work environment and improve the ability of nurses to provide care. This has become more of an imperative for this generation's nursing leaders to impact and improve nursing retention.

Nursing care in hospitals requires a framework of a professional nursing practice model, which is necessary as a foundation for care delivery. The professional nursing practice model needs to include a philosophy of nursing care and be based on a theory of practice that resonates with all of the nurses in the practice site. The nurses executive, working in partnership with the clinicians at the bedside, have a privileged opportunity to give substantive meaning to the philosophy of nursing and mission statement regarding the caring nature of nursing. "A well developed nursing conceptual framework that explicitly grounds nursing service and communicates the uniqueness of nursing as well as its connection to the other sectors of the health care system is the foundation for successful integration of theory into practice".[1] This article shares the results of a multiyear Health Resources and Services Administration (HRSA)–funded grant aimed at reducing work intensity for hospital nurses and creating a human caring environment in the acute care workplace.

BACKGROUND

Inova Health System is a not-for-profit, integrated health care system in northern Virginia that consists of five hospitals, two long-term care facilities, emergency care centers, and ambulatory services (including mental health and rehabilitation services) that serve a population of almost 2 million people. Each hospital and the continuum of care services has a chief nurse and a system chief nurse serves as the corporate representative of nursing at the highest executive level. The system chief nurse has responsibility for strategy and oversight of nursing practice, education, and research across the system.

As part of the nursing strategic planning process, Inova Health System chose to base its nursing practice on a nursing theory, and planned to

This work was supported by HRSA grant as part of the Division of Nursing and Bureau of Health Profession, Health Resources and Services Administration, Department of Health and Human Services, under grant number D66HP01383, Title VII, Enhancing Patient Care Delivery Systems.
Inova Health System, 2990 Telestar Court, Falls Church, VA 22042, USA
* 8515 Georgia Avenue, Silver Spring, MD 20910.
E-mail address: karen.drenkard@ana.org

Crit Care Nurs Clin N Am 20 (2008) 403–414
doi:10.1016/j.ccell.2008.08.008
0899-5885/08/$ – see front matter © 2008 Published by Elsevier Inc.

develop a professional nursing practice model that captured the essence of an American Nurses Credentialing Center (ANCC) Magnet Recognition Program hospital system. The nursing executive team went through a process of reviewing and examining the many nursing theories during a strategic planning process, and used shared governance strategies to engage staff in the decision-making process. Goals and measurement of the theory-based practice model included the improvement of nursing retention.

Through multiple focus groups and open forums, the decision was made to implement a human caring model of care. The philosophy of care was based on caring science, as conceptualized by Jean Watson.[2–4] Watson's[3] work included the identification of 10 caring factors, and has resulted in formal attention to "nursing theory as the disciplinary foundation for nursing science, education and practice." Watson[3] describes the process where any "nurse-patient encounter can be considered a caring occasion or caring moment, if it is conscious, intentional orientation based on humanistic values of kindness, empathy, concern and love." The nurse is described as the guide to the creation of a healing environment and the main therapeutic element in creating this environment for the patient.[5,6] In this caring science environment, "nursing contributes to the preservation of humanity and seeks to sustain caring in instances where it is threatened".[3]

The nursing leadership at Inova engaged the staff in creating a vision for the application of a human caring model. The staff nurses began the work of making the vision a reality. They quickly realized that to create a caring and healing environment, the care units needed to streamline "hassle factors"[7] and gain time back at the bedside to care more directly for patients. What began as a linear process of implementing a philosophy and model of care became a complex interactive process of work that took place over a 4-year time period.

The need to streamline work processes and provide nurses with more time to create a healing environment was a turning point for the work that was ahead. How could the nursing units implement a human caring model if the nurses were "too busy" to engage in the transformation? What strategies and opportunities did this present to the nursing leadership team?

OPPORTUNITIES IDENTIFIED

To create a healing environment, it was clear that the first step was to streamline some of the work processes, reduce work intensity, and eliminate some hassle factors for the nurses. Inova Health System applied for a HRSA grant as part of the Division of Nursing and Bureau of Health Profession, Health Resources and Services Administration, Department of Health and Human Services. Inova received a 4-year, $685,000 award to improve work processes so that a human caring model could be implemented across four hospitals. The project was called "Making Time for Caring." The chief nurse of the system was participating in a Robert Wood Johnson Executive Nurse Fellowship, and used funding that was allocated as part of the fellowship. The chief nurse executive applied these project funds for the dissemination of data and training materials to the nursing leadership community.

LITERATURE REVIEW

A review of the literature provides both methods and processes for engaging in decreasing work intensity to allow nurses more time actually to care for patients. One of the fundamental questions for nursing leadership is: "If nurses are able to streamline their work processes, how can one use that time positively to impact nursing practice?" This research project hypothesized that if work intensity was reduced, that would free up more time for the nurse to be present at the patients' side, allowing for more time for caring activities. Research is beginning to emerge that suggests that a core factor of a nurses' identity is the ability to respond to patient caring needs.[8] Constant interruptions and chaos in the care setting is a barrier to caring.

To assist nurses who are looking to redesign patient care delivery, the American Organization of Nurse Executives has identified key components of any research activities to examine work processes. They suggest evaluation components that include the determination and collection of baseline data to analyze productivity and then using that data to measure progress toward improvement of productivity.[9] Tools for work sampling are available to assist in this process.[10] Other multisite projects, such as Robert Wood Johnson Foundation's Transforming Care at the Bedside, support the assumption that taking the time to figure out what is wrong with care processes and then doing something about it is key to reducing work intensity and designing new processes of care.[11] Responses to streamlining the work of the nurse include innovative approaches to eliminating hunting and gathering activities, and simplifying documentation.[12] Beaudoin and Edgar[7] identified a methodology for assisting in the identification and elimination of hassle factors in an inpatient care unit, and began the link between these hassles and the human cost of inefficiency.

As a result of the literature review, and in response to staff feedback, it became clear that a two-phased approach is required to be successful in implementing a nursing professional practice model based on human caring theory. Phase I involved improving staff nurse satisfaction by decreasing work intensity. Phase II implemented a human caring environment with a goal of reducing nurse turnover and increasing satisfaction of both patients and nurses. By separating the effort into two distinct phases, nurses could see that their request for a streamlined work environment was being met before the implementation of a human caring model. This two-phased approach proved to be an effective strategy in gaining the support of the nursing staff who desired to have more time to interact with their patients, but perceived that they did not have the time to do so.

PURPOSE

The objective of the HRSA Nursing Retention Grant was to improve nurse satisfaction and retention by decreasing work intensity, streamlining cumbersome nursing processes, and creating a human caring environment in the workplace. The study engaged and involved staff nurses in the process.

STUDY DESIGN

This study was a quasiexperimental, between-subjects, naturalistic, longitudinal study on four pilot medical units and four surgical comparison units at Inova Health System. Inova Health System Institutional Review Board (IRB) approval was obtained. The unit of study was the patient care unit, rather than the individuals within the unit, and participants in the groups being compared were different people over time. The units were not randomly selected.

METHODS

The four medical units were chosen across four hospitals. Selection variables that were considered include leadership stability, current nursing vacancy and turnover rates, hours per patient day, and patient complexity. Four surgical units across the four hospitals were chosen as comparison units, and these units had no interventions during the study period. Preliminary data collection took place before any intervention, and included assessment of nursing turnover rates, patient and staff satisfaction scores, and RN satisfaction indicators from the National Database for Nursing Quality Indicators (NDNQI) data set. There were two phases of the study. Phase I was a process improvement

phase where work intensity was decreased on the pilot units resulting in more time available for staff nurses to provide direct patient care. Phase II was the implementation of caring processes on the pilot units, with premeasurement and postmeasurement of nurse satisfaction, nurse turnover, and patient satisfaction. No interventions except routine data collection occurred on the comparison units during the study time period. **Table 1** describes the protocol and timeline of the study.

Phase I: Decrease Work Intensity

Once the pilot units were chosen, groups of staff were brought together in work teams. These teams identified hassle factors that impacted the nurses' ability to complete work and resulted in interruptions and daily workflow inefficiencies. Each of the four units had to agree on the top four areas to address. Although there was some overlap in identified hassles, the group voted to come up with four improvement areas: (1) medication administration process, (2) admission-discharge-transfer process, (3) documentation process, and (4) communication process. Process and performance improvement methodologies were used to save nursing time.

Interventions for Phase I

For each of the four processes, cross-hospital teams worked to collect baseline data on the time each process took before any interventions. In addition, workflow diagrams were created. Once baseline data collection was completed, the teams worked together using quality improvement methodologies to develop interventions that would improve each work process. For each of the processes, the interventions and results are identified in **Table 2**. The process changes were implemented on each of the pilot units. Once the final data were collected and results showed improvement, all of the interventions were subsequently included in the strategic plan for the rest of the units across all of the hospital inpatient units. For example, the automated telephone messaging system for report was implemented across 75 inpatient units during year 3 of the study. The technology changes to documentation were also implemented across all of the hospitals and a plan for each unit to go wireless was put in place. Likewise, use of the pharmacy scanning system was initiated in all relevant patient care areas.

Results from Phase I

Data were collected from each of the pilot units and time was saved in each process area except in documentation, where total compliance scores increased (see **Table 2**). On completion of the

Table 1
Integrating human caring science into a professional nursing practice model: Inova Health System study design grid

Description of protocol	Year 1	Year 2	Year 3	Year 4	Year 5
Interventional group					
Preintervention phase					
Selection of study groups (pilot and control) based on variables	▓				
Phase I: decrease work intensity					
1. Work teams identify hassle factors	▓				
2. Work teams decide on four processes to address	▓				
Phase I: process improvement interventions					
1. Work teams collect baseline data on each of four processes (time wanding)	▓				
2. Work teams develop interventions to address four processes	▓				
3. Work teams pilot interventions to address four processes	▓				
4. Core process changes and implemented throughout Inova inpatient units		▓			
Phase II: creation of human caring environment					
1. Nurse caring behaviors identified for pilot testing			▓		
2. Integration of 10 caritas factors into practice model			▓		
3. Caring ambassadors selected on four interventional units			▓		
4. Ambassadors participate in 2-day caring science immersion education course: caring coaches designated			▓		
5. All staff members on interventional units participate in caring science educational sessions			▓		
6. Implementation of caritas factors into nursing practice			▓		
7. Implementation of caritas factors into all inpatient units			▓	▓	
8. Implementation of caritas factors on all outpatient and ambulatory care units					▓
Postintervention phase					
Quantitative data collection	▓	▓			
Caring Assessment Tool Version II		▓			
Caring Factor Survey		▓			
Healthcare Environment Survey		▓			
NDNQI Nurse Satisfaction Survey	▓	▓			
Inova internal turnover and vacancy rates	▓	▓	▓	▓	
Qualitative data collection					
Focus groups					
Comparison group					
Preintervention phase					
Selection of study groups based on variables	▓				
Phase I: routine Inova data collection					
No targeted interventions; routine organizational processes	▓	▓	▓	▓	
Post-intervention phase					
Routine Inova data collection and organizational processes	▓	▓	▓	▓	▓

Table 2
Improved work processes

Hassle Factor and Process	Identified Interventions to Save Time	Results in Time Savings
Medication administration process *Hassle*: "Time for pharmacy to get orders was too long, resulting in delays"	Piloted use of a medication order scanning process to speed time that physician order arrived in pharmacy.	Med Order Scanners streamlined the process from 30–60 minutes per order sheet.
Admission/discharge/transfer process *Hassle*: "Time to admit patient was too long"	Piloted use of an admission nurse, sole job to admit, discharge and transfer patients on medical unit. Also assisted in "hunting and gathering" activities related to patient admission, including beginning nursing care interventions. Greeted and oriented patient, obtained equipment, documented vital signs and patient history, performed and documented initial patient assessment.	Using an admissions nurse reduced the average time to admit a patient from 75.93 minutes to 56.13 minutes; resulting in 18.2-minute decrease in time for admission.
Documentation process *Hassle*: "Paper documentation was too redundant"	Automated on-line documentation system for multiple forms on medical unit, use of "computers on wheels" to facilitate point of service documentation.	Improved compliance with documentation from 85%–98%.
Communication process *Hassle*: "Time spent on report was too long, hunting and gathering for report supplies was a waste of time"	Piloted "VoiceCare" system, a telephone voicemail system for report, allowing for prerecorded patient history to be repeated each shift.	VoiceCare expedited shift change communication by 3.6 minutes per patient per report, or more than 10 minutes per patient.

process improvement pilots, the nursing satisfaction survey was redistributed to the staff on the four medical units. The nurses' perception of having sufficient time to attend to the emotional and psychosocial needs of the patients improved 16.2% and a 13.1% improvement was noted in having sufficient time for direct patient care as a result of changes in the admission process.

There was improvement in nurse satisfaction of the role of the admission nurse, which is one element of improving work intensity. The nurses' perception of benefit of the admission role as a result of the pilot was a score of 5.67 overall benefit on a scale of 1 to 6. As a result of all of the process improvement work that was done, core process changes were made to the pilot units and then spread throughout Inova Health System inpatient units during the course of years 2 and 3. Once the pilot units had completed the process improvement changes, Phase II of the studies began.

Phase II: Creation of a Human Caring Environment

Phase II included the development and implementation of a human caring work environment based on the work of theorist Dr. Jean Watson.[13] In Watson's theory, the patient is an equal partner with health care providers to optimize wellness physically, emotionally, and spiritually. The objective in this phase was to improve staff nurse satisfaction and turnover rates by providing the nurse time to practice the art of nursing in a caring and healing environment within an acute care setting. A review of the literature led to the discovery of caring behaviors that were considered for the pilot.[14–19] Watson worked with Inova Health System to design the translation of the Human Caring processes into key interventions for the study. The interventions were also based on the literature that described the importance of nurse caring behaviors in acute care settings[20–23] and throughout the continuum of care.[24] Finfgeld-Connett[18] share that a work environment conducive to caring is necessary for caring to occur, and the environmental factors include improvements in coworker support, teamwork, supportive management, learning experiences, and adequate time to care for patients. Behaviors that were well documented in the literature[18] that constitute caring include attentive listening, making eye contact, touching, offering verbal reassurance, being physically and mindfully present, centering on the patient, being emotionally open and available, and taking cultural differences into consideration. Activities include listening, providing information, encouraging expressions of concern, and helping cope with difficult situations. All of these were considered as the interventions were designed to create a healing and caring environment in the study.

In addition, effort was dedicated to determining appropriate measurement tools based on the literature review.[2,25,26] The translation of Watson's caritas processes into shared language that was developed by Westlake Hospital nursing staff in Melrose, Illinois, was used to help the Inova staff understand that caring is a process.[18] Permission was granted to use the Westlake description of Watson's caring processes throughout the Inova Health System pilot.

The 10 caring (caritas) factors described in a simplified interpretation developed by Westlake Hospital, Melrose, Illinois, are based on Watson's theory and are included in **Box 1**.

Box 1
Translation of Watson's caritas processes: caring factors

1. Practice loving kindness
2. Instill faith and hope
3. Nurture individual spiritual beliefs and practices
4. Developing helping-trusting relationships
5. Promote and accept the expression of positive and negative feelings
6. Use creative scientific problem solving methods for decision-making
7. Perform teaching and learning that addresses the individual needs and learning styles
8. Create a healing environment for the physical and spiritual self that respects human dignity
9. Assist with physical, emotional, and spiritual human needs
10. Allow room for miracles to take place

Courtesy of Westlake Hospital, Melrose, Illinois.

Work teams on Inova's pilot units worked together to determine key factors of human caring and interventions were developed and then implemented on the pilot units. The interventions included several key efforts at educating and coaching the nursing staff in the implementation of caring activities. Ambassadors on each of the four pilot units were chosen to be the champions of the care changes. These ambassadors participated in a 2-day immersion course led by Watson and Dr. Janet Quinn, where the human caring theory was fully explained and the ambassadors were trained in centering techniques, intentionality exercises, and being more fully present with patients. Training included intentionality or "being in the moment" with patients, caring connection or taking time to care and connect with each patient, and reflection and celebration or honoring the power that lies in service to others based on the 10 caring factors.

The ambassadors were also cultivated into "caring coaches" and were encouraged to develop monitoring capability on their care units. For example, they learned to collect data and give feedback to staff as they served as a role model for caring behaviors in daily work. After the ambassadors were trained, a curriculum was developed for all of the staff on the pilot units. This curriculum content included intentionality and centering techniques (being "in the moment" with patients); breathing techniques that helped to decrease stress and improve concentration for both staff and patients; caring connections (taking time each day to care and connect with each patient); reflection and celebration of positive events through the ritual of hand washing in the care area; participating and leading caring circles to recenter thoughts around the patient; creation of a caring lounge on each patient care unit for nurses to retreat to find quiet space for recentering and reflection; and monitoring, observing, and evaluating peer activities.

Some examples of practice changes that were implemented and evaluated include the following:

Nurses spent up to 5 minutes each shift with each patient focusing on authentically being present with the patient and interacting with them in this connected space. This time allowed the patient to be a partner in care and helped the nurse understand the patients' perception of need for caring. The nurse spent time in a way that conveyed concern and respect, being present with the patient, face to face, at the eye level of the patient. The nurse used touch as appropriate and was able to relate to the patient on a very human level.

- Nurses used the time spent for hand washing and transformed it into a ritual of thanks for having the ability and privilege to care for each patient. For many the hand washing time became a time to reflect on closure and completion of the human caring experience between patient encounters.
- Nurses used motivational signs that were hung over each sink and magnets placed outside the door of each room to help them focus on being intentional in their work before each patient interaction. Each nurse stopped before entering the room to pause, read the message of hope and healing, and become centered on the patient encounter.
- Nurses placed posters on each unit with the 10 caring factors in a large display for patients, families, and staff members to be able to visualize the commitment to caring behaviors.
- On some units, the nursing staff decided to decrease the lighting level, which impacted the noise level on the pilot units.
- All of the pilot units created a centering lounge. Staff used this lounge as a place to center and learn about human caring. Some units called it their nursing "sanctuary" where staff could practice their breathing techniques. Peer coaches identified staff that were stressed and encouraged them to take a break in the centering lounge as a way to recenter around the patients.

At Inova Health System, the goal continues to be the creation of an intentional environment within the hospital setting that addresses the needs of the nurse, the patient, and colleagues. Training interventions began at the end of year 2 and continued through year 5.

Results from Phase II

Measurement tools Baseline data were collected from several sources, including the review of tools that have been especially developed to measure the impact of human caring activities on nurses and patients.[25–27] For this research study, several measurement surveys were used. To understand better the patient's perception of caring based on Watson's theory of caring, Inova used the Caring Assessment Tool (CAT) Version II developed by Duffy and coworkers[27] at Catholic University. The CAT II tool has established content validity and reliability when used in an acute care setting. The

Caring Factor Survey measured the impact of the 10 caring processes on patient's perception of caring by the nurse. The Caring Factor Survey was developed by John Nelson[15] and has only been used to test the psychometric properties of the tool (Cronbach's alpha 0.97). Both the CAT II and the Caring Factor Survey measurement tools are based on the caritas processes, which are concepts of caring based on the theory and work of Watson.

To evaluate nurse satisfaction, the Healthcare Environment Survey (HES) developed by Nelson was used.[15] The HES is a valid and reliable (Cronbach's alpha 0.96) 86-item instrument used to obtain staff members' perception of the work environment, including relationships with coworkers, unit manager, physicians, and nurses; professional patient care; autonomy; staffing and scheduling; executive leadership; learning opportunities; organizational rewards; pride in the organization; intent to stay; and workload.

Other data collection included review of Inova's employee opinion survey and the NDNQI RN satisfaction survey that was being collected at each hospital. In addition, turnover data were collected and evaluated during year 4 of the study.

Patient perception of caring Results of the CAT II measured patient's perception of caring, preintervention and postintervention. In the pilot group, there were 134 patients in the pre–data collection and 155 patients postcaring interventions. Data were also collected on the comparison units, which consisted of 141 patients in the pregroup and 127 in the postintervention group. When compared with the preintervention group, patients on both pilot and comparison units reported more satisfaction with care at postintervention. Score differences, however, were not statistically significant for either group (using an alpha of .05). On the pilot units, scores increased 0.12 points on a scale of 1 to 7.

Patient satisfaction Inova Health System uses Professional Research Consultants (PRC) to measure inpatient hospital satisfaction data. During this study, the investigators used the data from PRC to evaluate patient satisfaction. PRC data are valid and reliable across hundreds of hospitals across the United States. The tool measures scores of percent "excellent." Data comparison on the pilot units from 2005 (preintervention) to 2006 (postintervention) during the time of the caring protocols showed improvement in overall patient satisfaction (**Fig. 1**). The percent ranked excellent improved on the pilot units from 9.9% to 79.2% precaring interventions to 57.6% to 98.7% postcaring interventions. Improvements were seen in each of the pilot units.

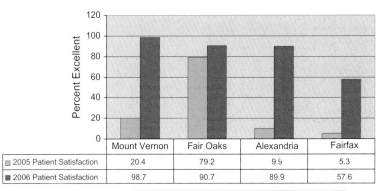

Fig. 1. Comparison of patient satisfaction 2005 (preintervention) compared with 2006 (postintervention) on human caring pilot units; measures percent ranked "excellent" on Professional Research Consultants data collection tool.

	Mount Vernon	Fair Oaks	Alexandria	Fairfax
2005 Patient Satisfaction	20.4	79.2	9.9	5.3
2006 Patient Satisfaction	98.7	90.7	89.9	57.6

Nurse satisfaction In November 2004, the HES was distributed to 621 nurses at Inova Health System for the baseline assessment. The "caring protocol" had not been implemented on any unit, but several staff had attended introductory classes at the time of the baseline measurement. One hundred and sixty-five nurses from the pilot units returned the survey (a 52% response rate) and 113 nurses from the comparison units returned the survey (a 37% response rate). Combined, 278 nurses returned the survey (a 45% response rate). Results of the 277 usable surveys were analyzed using various statistical methods. These were considered the predata set.

In February 2006, the HES survey was repeated. A total of 578 staff participated in the sample with 291 staff responding (50% response rate). There were 131 staff who responded to the HES at both premeasurement and postmeasurement (approximately 23% of the staff). Responses of those who participated in both measurements were used within the final paired *t*-test, comparing the changes of the postintervention scores with the baseline scores. Respondents to the HES were asked to rank their level of satisfaction using a Likert-type scale (ranging from one to seven, strongly dissatisfied to strongly satisfied, respectively) on workforce environmental variables.

The results revealed no significant differences in demographics over time, indicating stability on the unit. The interaction effect of the pilot comparison group that was statistically significant at the 0.05 level (**Table 3**) were the HES total score, relationship with coworkers subscale score, and workload perception subscale score.

Other improvements that were noted, but were not statistically significant, included relationship with physicians, pride in the organization, promotional opportunities being present, and improved relationships with other nurses.

Nurse satisfaction: National Database for Nursing Quality Indicators data The NDNQI offers an RN satisfaction survey that is conducted annually for those hospitals opting to participate. The question that the study compared was the Nurse-Nurse Interaction score on NDNQI: "Do nurses help each other, feel at home on the unit, is there teamwork, are nurses friendly to each other?" Comparing the scores of 2005 before intervention and 2006

Table 3
Positive improvement in health care environment survey subscores postintervention of the caring protocol

Variable	Change Score Combined Pilot Units	Change Score Combined Comparison Units
Health care environmental survey total score	0.09[a]	0.05
Workload	0.21[a]	−0.17
Relationship with coworkers	0.21[a]	−0.16
Promotional opportunities	0.10	0.02
Pride in the organization	0.07	0.02

[a] Statistically significant at 0.05 level.

postintervention on the four medical pilot units, three out of four units improved to a level considered "high satisfaction" by the survey guidelines (**Table 4**).

Turnover and vacancy rates of registered nurses on pilot units These indicators were by far the most difficult to analyze, because there are many reasons that RNs choose to leave or resign from a care unit. Nonetheless, a comparison of the pilot units during the time period of the study and ongoing has revealed a lower rate of turnover and vacancy, and a decrease of vacancy and turnover rates over time. The primary driver for RN turnover could not be determined, although the relationship with patients remained the nurses' number one source of job satisfaction. **Table 5** shows a sample of one unit's tracking of retention during the 6-month pilot time period of human caring practice interventions. Although improvement was noted compared with the comparison units, there was inconsistency and no statistically significant trends when this was studied across all of the pilot units and comparison units for the health system.

Qualitative data During the study time period, opportunities to engage staff and hear feedback in focus groups about what was working and what did not work helped to guide the process of education and coaching on the units. Focus groups were held, and surveys were administered that allowed nurses to share their stories about what it was like to practice nursing in an environment where caring processes were encouraged and expected. The following statements capture the essence of the feedback with themes of nurses feeling able to care for themselves, to care for each other as coworkers, and to increase their intentional care for patients.

- "By starting with the present from within me, and coming with a good heart, I am able to deliver the best care I ever thought possible."
- "I am able to take more time to clear my mind and take time to focus on each issue."
- "I am in the process of ordering my private world. I now have the learning tools to cope with situations in a positive way; now I am learning to be in the present."
- "Because we are all doing this together, I know that my patients are going to get great care from my coworkers too."
- "I have felt a renewal of spirituality, love, and caring energy that allows me to care for my patients."
- "This work enhances the caring spirit, which I try to administer with every patient."
- "I gave one of our patients a brief massage the day before yesterday. She truly loved it. It gave her some respite from her physical and mental suffering. Were it not for caritas, I would not have even considered this."
- " I have been a nurse about 2 years now, and I had been feeling frustrated because I was not able to spend enough time interacting with my patients. I was actually thinking of leaving nursing because I was so discouraged. By being able to have the time to implement the human caring interventions, my perspective has changed and I have the support from my coworkers and nursing leadership to spend time with my patients. It has made all the difference for me, and I cannot imagine being anything but a nurse."

LIMITATIONS OF THE STUDY

Limitations of the study include no random assignment of control and intervention units, which may have led to a systematic bias. Not all of the variables could be manipulated and the caring interventions could not be controlled as the only variables, making it difficult to attribute cause and effect inferences. The long time frame of the study meant that other changes occurred on the care units over the 4-year time period, such as changes in leadership and opening and closing

Table 4
National Database for Nursing Quality Indicators Nurse-Nurse Interaction score

Unit	2005 Score	2006 Score
Inova Fairfax Hospital Tower 8 Medicine	71.25	72.39
Inova Alexandria Hospital Unit 23 Medicine	63.54	72.72
Inova Fair Oaks Hospital 4 New Medicine	61.91	60.86
Inova Mount Vernon Hospital 3B Medicine	49.27	57.65

"Do nurses help each other, feel at home on the unit, is there teamwork, are nurses friendly to each other?" Pilot units' comparison between 2005 and 2006.
Scale: <40, low satisfaction; 40–60, moderate satisfaction; >60, high satisfaction.
Shaded scores indicate improvement.

| Table 5 | | | | | | | |
| Example of retention results | | | | | | | |
Units	Jan	Feb	Mar	Apr	May	June	July
Control	100	100	77.8	83.3	86.7	77.8	81
Pilot	100	100	100	83.3	86.7	88.9	100

Inova Mount Vernon Hospital Comparison versus pilot units percent registered nurse retention rates, January–July 2006. Includes voluntary and involuntary terminations during time period studied.

of new units. In addition, there may have been a double Hawthorne effect[28] because some of the surgical units became aware of the changes occurring on the pilot medical units because those units were receiving a lot of attention over time. As a result, causal links and cause and effect inferences need to be made with care.

MOVING BEYOND THE STUDY

Creation of Inova's Human Caring professional practice model has continued beyond the four pilot units. During 2007, education sessions were created and four to six staff nurses from each of the 75 inpatient units attended special sessions to be educated in the practice changes for creating a healing and caring environment. Over 1000 RNs were trained. Each unit received $1000 to create a healing lounge area and staff members were very creative in transforming small spaces into special areas for centering. A toolkit was distributed to each of the remaining 70 inpatient units. The toolkit consisted of posters with the display of the 10 caritas processes for the unit; magnets for enhancing intentionality to be placed on the door jams; brochures (education and information); caritas cards (used for reminder of the caring processes); pins to recognize staff who had attended education sessions; inspirational quotes with suction cups (to be placed in hand washing areas); and the CD "human caring meditations" for use in centering during a shift.

During 2008, the Inova Human Caring model was implemented in the ambulatory and outpatient centers. Educational sessions were held during first and second quarter, with over 200 staff attending from multidisciplinary backgrounds. In addition, the caring processes and interventions are now included in the Inova infrastructure. These include the development of a philosophy of care based on Human Caring Theory, inclusion of the caring processes into orientation for new staff members, integration of caring processes into the job profile and job descriptions of RN 1 to 4 categories and the annual competencies and annual evaluation, the development of a nursing model of care based on caring processes, development of a recognition program called the Caritas Awards, quarterly workshops included in the learning network and education programming, a special internal Web site devoted to human caring activities, and most recently the introduction of a Human Caring Research Internship Program. This work has also led to the development of an evolving Inova Model of Care based on caring processes, which is in the final stages of completion. These foundational elements are critical to ensuring that the human caring work continues and that the caring processes are encouraged in an integrated manner across all hospitals and care settings within Inova.

SUMMARY

The unique contribution of this study is that it involved two distinct phases of work to improve nursing care at the bedside. Although the ultimate goal was to implement a human caring philosophy, the staff nurses in the practice environment shared their perspective about inefficient work processes and hassle factors in care. Only by improving those processes first could the integrative nursing work of caring and healing be implemented. Quality improvement and work process redesign should be a core project activity in every patient care area, with ongoing efforts at improving efficiency and freeing up the nurse to be more present with patients.

Although studies are emerging that describe how nurses are spending their time with non–value added tasks and activities, such as hunting and gathering for supplies,[29] very few have suggested what the nurse should do with the time saved when processes are improved. Streamlining work processes can gain time back at the bedside, giving nurses the opportunity to establish a more meaningful, caring connection with patients. This enhanced ability to provide nursing care in a healing and caring environment has led to greater work fulfillment, a sense of belonging, commitment to the care unit, and improved morale. Findings from this study show that nurses are very willing to enhance their therapeutic relationships with patients and feel more satisfied when they make that connection.

It is incumbent on nursing practice leaders, from bedside nurse to chief nurse, to make space for quality improvement projects that improve care efficiency so that the nurse can redirect time toward caring encounters with patients. Caring interventions should be well described, taught, and coached. The caring interventions described in this study are not separate activities, but rather integrated activities to be woven throughout the day, or the visit, or the encounter. Watson describes this as caring as transpersonal relationship between the nurse and the patient. This is a special kind of human care relationship, a union with a high regard for the whole person and their being in the world.[16] Whitmer and coworkers[17] describes the need for caring as especially evident in the critical care environment, where nurses face the dilemma of a lack of time to complete nursing tasks and provide comfort.

This study suggests that making time for caring is a necessary step to maximize the nursing practice contribution. If time is saved, then the redirection of that time to care processes that allow the nurse to serve as an agent of healing at the bedside is realized. Being able to create a caring environment is a privileged opportunity for nursing leadership.[1] Understanding nursing as a caring science and the ability to create a caring culture, where the processes of care are grounded in connection with the patients, is the role of every nurse. The ability of nurses to serve as role models so that caring processes and interventions are valued over simple task completion ensures that the next generation of nurses has job fulfillment and that patients are cared for in a holistic manner.

ACKNOWLEDGMENTS

The author acknowledges the contribution of Gene Rigotti, RN, MSN, and Jean Watson, PhD, RN, ANC, BC, FAAN, to the content of the article.

REFERENCES

1. Boykin A, Schoenhofer S. The role of nursing leadership in creating caring environments in health care delivery systems. Nurs Adm Q 2001;25(3):1–7.
2. Watson J. Nursing: the philosophy and science of caring. Colorado (CO): University Press of Colorado; 1985.
3. Watson J. Watson's theory of human caring and subjective living experiences: carative factors/caritas processes as a disciplinary guide to the professional nursing practice. Texto and Contexto Enfermagem, Florianopolis. Brazil: University of Santa Catarina; 2007. p. 129–35.
4. Watson J, Smith MC. Caring science and the science of unitary human beings: a trans-theoretical discourse for nursing knowledge development. J Adv Nurs 2002;37(5):452–61.
5. McCormack B, McCance TV. Development of a framework for person-centered nursing: nursing theory and concept development or analysis. J Adv Nurs 2006;56(5):472–9.
6. Sumner J. Caring in nursing: a different interpretation. J Adv Nurs 2001;35(6):926–32.
7. Beaudoin LE, Edgar L. Hassles: their importance to nurses' quality of work life. Nurs Econ 2003;21(3): 106–13.
8. Fagerstrom L. The dialectic tension between being and not being a good nurse. Nurs Ethics 2006; 13(6):622–31.
9. Patient care delivery and work design, pdf manual, May 2003. Available at: www.aone.org/aone/docs/ hwe_excellence_initiatives.pdf. Accessed June 29, 2008.
10. Urden LD, Rooder JL. Work sampling: a decision-making tool for determining resources and work redesign. J Nurs Adm 1997;27(9):34–41.
11. Viney M, Batcheller J, Hourston S, et al. Transforming care at the bedside: designing new care systems in an age of complexity. J Nurs Care 2006; 21(2):143–50.
12. Fuller J. Regarding work intensity, less is more. Nurs Manage 2007;28(5):12.
13. Watson J. Caring theory as an ethical guide to administrative and clinical practices. JONAS Healthc Law Ethics Regul 2006;8(3):87–93.
14. Carter LC, Nelson JL, Sievers BA, et al. Exploring a culture of caring. Nurs Adm Q 2008;32(1):57–63.
15. Persky GL, Nelson J, Watson J, et al. Creating a profile of a nurse effective in caring. Nurs Adm Q 2008; 32(1):15–20.
16. Rexroth R, Davidhizar R. Caring: utilizing the Watson theory to transcend culture. Health Care Manag (Frederick) 2003;22(4):295–304.
17. Whitmer M, Hurst S, Stakder K, et al. Caring in the curing environment: the implementation of a grieving cart in the ICU. Journal of Hospice and Palliative Nursing 2007;9(6):329–33.
18. Finfgeld-Connett D. Meta-synthesis of caring in nursing. J Clin Nurs 2008;17:196–204.
19. Hemsley MS, Glass N, Watson J. Taking the eagles' view: using Watson's conceptual model to investigate the extraordinary and transformative experiences of nurse healers. Holist Nurs Pract 2006; 20(2):85–94.
20. Baldursdottir G, Jonsdottir H. The importance of nurse caring behaviors as perceived by patient receiving care in an emergency department. Heart Lung 2002;31(1):67–75.

21. Wang CH. Knowing and approaching hope as human experience: implications for the medical-surgical nurse. Medsurg Nurs 2000;9(4):189–93.

22. Chung LY, Wong FK, Chan MF. Relationship of nurses' spirituality to their understanding and practice of spiritual care. J Adv Nurs 2007;58(2):158–70.

23. Rosenberg S. Utilizing the language of Jean Watson's caring theory within a computerized clinical documentation system. Comput Inform Nurs 2006; 24(1):53–6.

24. Owens RA. The caring behaviors of the home health nurse and influence on medication adherence. Home Healthcare Nurse 2006;24(8):517–26.

25. Cossette S, Cote JK, Pepin J, et al. A dimensional structure of nursing patient interactions from a caring perspective: refinement of the Caring Nurse-Patient Interactino Scale (CNPI- short scale). J Adv Nurs 2006;55(2):198–214.

26. Beck CT. Quantitative measurement of caring. J Adv Nurs 1999;30(1):24–32.

27. Duffy J, Hoskins L, Seifert RF. Dimensions of caring: psychometric evaluation of the caring assessment tool. ANS Adv Nurs Sci 2007;30(3):235–45.

28. Polit DF, Beck CT, Hungler BP. Essentials of nursing research, methods, appraisal, and utilization. 5th edition. Baltimore (MD): Lippincott; 2001.

29. Hendrich A, Chow MP, Skierczynski BA, et al. A 36 hospital time and motion study: how do medical surgical nurses spend their time? The Permanente Journal 2008;3(12):25–33.

Cultural Competence Models in Nursing

G. Rumay Alexander, EdD, RN

KEYWORDS

- Cultural competence • Cultural competency models
- Diversity • Health care delivery • Theory of change
- Theoretic frameworks

Of all the forms of inequality, injustice in health care is the most shocking and inhumane.
Dr. Martin Luther King, Jr.

According to the American Organization of Nurse Executives' 2007 Position Statement and Guiding Principles for Diversity in Health Care Organizations, globalization, new technology, war, threats of bioterrorism, and ecosystem imbalances represent only the beginning of America's heightened awareness of movement between cultures and countries and the pervasive effects this has unleashed.[1,2] Even with the acknowledgment of these inconvenient truths, there is undeniable evidence that highlights continued acts of denial, resistance, and other desperate human actions to control that which is uncontrollable. Of all the issues, those related to demographic changes and the voices of difference seem to present the most struggle. Modern America is home to millions of immigrants. Today's workforce is a reflection of the considerable mix of cultures, ages, new family configurations, religions, and races. Diversity in its many forms will be a part of the future and requires new social interactions, societal expectations, and mandates. Accordingly, it is time to get serious about diversity.

Historically for the United States, the education of health care providers has focused on the demographic majority that is European-American. Despite growing evidence of the significant effect of psychosocial and behavioral factors in the onset, presentation, and prognosis of many illnesses,[3] a biomedical model remains dominant in medical practice. In a country with growing population diversity, care nevertheless has been increasingly standardized (and not necessarily in compliance with practice guidelines) rather than customized to individual patient and family needs or preferences. The current health care workforce has not been adequately prepared or educated to care or work with persons of the nonmajority culture in anything other than in a dominating, overseer type role. Such approaches have added insult to injury (often referred to as "microaggressions") and rendered the provider or the care environment countereffective in providing optimum care. Calls have been issued on providing culturally appropriate care and understanding the context for its provision. Moreover, compelling arguments and policy development to hold providers of care accountable and to train the workforce have been called for by the US Department of Health and Human Services Office of Minority Health's Culturally and Linguistically Appropriate Standards, the Joint Commission on Accreditation of Healthcare Organizations, and such landmark reports as The Sullivan Report: Missing in Action in 2006 and the Institute of Medicine's Unequal Treatment: Confronting Racial and Ethnic Disparities in Healthcare in 2002.[4–7] The link between cultural competency and patient safety caused by the dimensionality in presentation of patient's symptoms and the need for providers to be familiar with such dimensionality (if they are to intervene and respond in a timely manner) is also getting greater attention.

Growth of traditionally underrepresented ethnic minority groups and the aging of the population pose a dilemma for the country and its systems. Official definitions of the social system call for equality, whereas many of the informal features of this system demonstrate inequality. The pursuit

School of Nursing, CB 7460, University of North Carolina at Chapel Hill, Chapel Hill, NC 27599–7460, USA
E-mail address: rumay@email.unc.edu

Crit Care Nurs Clin N Am 20 (2008) 415–421
doi:10.1016/j.ccell.2008.08.012

of happiness, justice, and liberty continues to be available to some and withheld from others at the expense of all. Statutory reality in the United States has not caught up with constitutional morality and racial apartheid exists in state statutes. Efforts to build "a more perfect union" have not been perfect and they continue to plague this country. Nowhere is that more evident than when looking closely at the issues of providing cultural and linguistically appropriate health care services.

This article provides heuristic interpretation on cultural competency frameworks that can be used in clinical practice to deliver the care needed for today's culturally diverse patient population. Two frameworks are presented: the American Organization of Nurse Executives Guiding Principles for Diversity in Healthcare Organizations, and the adapted shifting perspectives model (**Fig. 1**).

MIRROR, MIRROR ON THE WALL

Culture, like genetics, not only has a group definition, but also an individual expression. Culture is an individual concept, a group phenomenon, and an organizational reality. It is shared, learned, dynamic, and evolutionary. The construct of culture also implies a dynamic, nested systems perspective that goes beyond discussions of race and ethnicity to include diverse subcultures. Subcultures include communities of interest (ie, religious denominations, fraternities, sororities, the elderly, persons with disabilities, breast cancer survivors). Each individual, family, and community represents a unique blend of overlapping and intersecting cultural elements in which the whole is greater than the sum of the parts. Understanding complexities of culture from the perspective of providers and recipients of care is critical because culture pervades all aspects of health care and all aspects of life. To say that this is not an easy task is an understatement, because "culture hides much more than it reveals, and strangely enough, what it hides, it hides most effectively from its own participants."[8] Culture does this silently at an

unconscious but powerful level as evidenced by the following musings:

- Racial bias and racism exist and function at all levels. No institution, system, or person is exempt. It threatens personal identity. Whether maligned, benign, or just plain misguided, it hurts all Americans, male and female; rich and poor; white, black, or Native American.
- There are two Americas and two systems of health care. According to former Surgeon General Dr. David Satcher, "if you want high quality health care it's good to speak English, be white and rich." (Dr. David Satcher, workshop, 2006)
- White privilege gives white students, white patients, and white colleagues in the workforce an edge over those who are nonwhite. Research reveals that whites fast track early to executive levels, whereas the nonmajority stays much longer in middle management. The reason for such outcomes is the lack of mentoring candidates of color receive.[8]
- Difference is seen and labeled as a problem. Teamwork and conformity are considered to be synonymous terms and are often used interchangeably. The aversion to differences is the result and the environments of care, education, and work are viewed as unwelcoming by those who are different from the majority.
- A commercial ethos exists in a social system.
- Abuse of power is growing in prevalence and practice, destroying the self-esteem of demographic populations that will be available and needed in the future.

Shaping the preferred future requires models or frameworks, leadership, political will, resilience, common sense, uncommon courage, and courageous dialog. Individuals and organizations can only change how they act if they are aware of their beliefs and assumptions. Examining assumptions about what is civil and any characteristics that hold people hostage to circumstances and situations over which they have no control is time well spent. In doing so, the level of self-awareness is raised, and in self-awareness begins the cultural competence journey. All encounters are cultural encounters and at the point of patient provider interaction three cultural encounters (the patient's, the provider's, and the organization's) occur simultaneously. This basic understanding is essential to producing the changes in thinking that

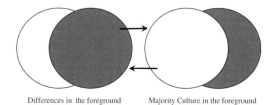

Differences in the foreground   Majority Culture in the foreground

Fig. 1. The shifting perspectives model of chronic illness. (*Adapted from* Paterson BL. The shifting perspectives model of chronic illness. J Nurs Scholarsh 2001;33:23; with permission.)

are necessary for respecting the culture of those under care.

UNDERSTANDING BY DESIGN

For the kind of understanding that makes for transformation at the human level, there must be a change in the "heart" and the "psychologic skin" of the environment. One of the most effective strategies for managing complexity, change, and establishing accountability is for system stakeholders to develop a clear link between their ideas and the strategies they intend to put into place.[9] The result of an idea is never separate from its source. Furthermore, thoughts always reveal themselves in behavior.

The theory of change articulates the underlying beliefs and assumptions that guide and are believed to be critical for producing the desired change or enable a person to meet the needs being addressed. A theory of change establishes clear links or connections between a system's mission and goals and actual outcomes. It is an approach that provides a way to make the the de facto system visible and subject to thoughtful examination.[9]

According to Hernandez and Hodges,[10] there are three types of theories of change: (1) recorded theory (conceptualization); (2) expressed theory (operationalization); and (3) active theory (implementation). The first two are future oriented and the third is present oriented. Cultural competency encompasses all three. Edge[11] further elucidates that competency is "the ability to function effectively and to appreciate the gifts of those who look different, who were raised differently than we were." The core elements of the theory (the population context, the strategies to be used, and the goals or desired outcomes) are laid out so that the relationships between the three can be understood and conveyed. When this theory of change is applied to cultural competence, for example, a clear picture is outlined for the stakeholders such that cultural competence is easily recognizable wherever and whenever it is in use. Developing cultural competence happens by design and intention, not by default.

CULTURAL COMPETENCE: KNOWING IT WHEN SEEING IT

Some see cultural competence as a process, others as an outcome, and then there are those who see it as the skill that enables one to embrace diversity.[12] Anyone who desires to engage in such deliberate learning finds that reflection, critical thinking, and active participation in their learning

is required. Without a doubt, cultural competencies are specific cognitive, affective, and psychomotor skills that are necessary for the facilitation of cultural congruence between provider and patient. Cultural competence is not an end point; an intention of eventual mastery is not possible. Approaches to cultural competence acquisition can be categorized as fact-centered or attitude- and skill-centered.[13] The attitude- and skill-centered approach represents a universal approach to cultural competence that enhances communication skills and emphasizes the particular sociocultural context of individuals. Like cultural competence training approaches, cross-cultural health programs and initiatives at the organizational level often fall into one of two categories: programs that focus on specific population groups, or health conditions and programs that address overall organizational cultural competence. The fact that it does not neatly fit into one of the types gives a plausible explanation for why there are so many frameworks in existence. Nine cultural, theoretic frameworks,[14–23] one meta-analysis,[14] and various evolving frameworks[24–27] are referenced in the literature.

Recognizing that both nursing care and culturally competent care are patient-centered care, the American Organization of Nurse Executives developed guiding principles for diversity in health care organizations in 2005 and updated these in 2007 (**Box 1**). These strategic and salient principles not only teach and raise the level of awareness for cultural competence; they also provide a means for evaluating the achievement of inclusive initiatives.

MODELS: SIX DEGREES OF INSPIRATION

The purpose of any model is to guide or inspire the user toward the preferred future as viewed by the model's creator. To provide greater clarity about the use of models, an acronym has been created that operationalizes what models do to enhance the user's understanding (**Box 2**).

In chronic illness, a helpful framework known as the "shifting perspectives model" is used. It was derived from a metasynthesis of 292 qualitative research studies on the perspectives of chronic illness.[13] The model shows living with chronic illness as an ongoing, continually shifting process in which people experience a complex dialectic between themselves and their "world." The shifting perspective model not only has application for chronic illness, but it also has value in cultural competence.

The chronic illness experience is depicted in the shifting perspective model as ever changing

---

Box 1
American Organization of Nurse Executives Guiding Principles for Diversity in Health Care Organizations

The following principles are intended to guide the nurse leader in achieving a diverse workforce by becoming an advocate for resources to implement and support a diversity program, encouraging a commitment to education, and leading diversity research initiatives that are based on performance improvement outcomes.

Guiding principle 1: Health care organizations will strive to develop internal and external resources to meet the needs of the diverse patient and workforce populations served

- Designate fiscal resources to develop programs and policies to meet the needs of diverse patient populations served.
- Establish system processes to ensure the needs of all patient populations are met.
- Include members from the local community with diverse backgrounds in organizational planning processes.
- Educate the community on the importance of collecting data, including patient and workforce race, ethnicity, and primary language spoken, for use in improving patient safety and quality.
- Develop processes and policies to ensure that non-English speaking and limited English proficiency patients will be assured of access to interpretive services and written translated patient education materials and documents.
- Implement processes to promote both the consistency of quality of care across various patient populations, and a balance in demographics between the patient and the workforce populations.
- Execute employment recruitment plans and strategies to attract a workforce that is reflective of the populations served.
- Train staff members in the importance of understanding the diversity of the patient population served and provision of culturally competent care.
- Support staff members in obtaining training and education in health care interpretation.

Guiding principle 2: Health care organizations will aim to establish a healthful practice/work environment that is reflective of diversity through a commitment to inclusivity, tolerance, and governance structures

- Encourage the employment of diverse groups of health care professionals.
- Actively involve all people in a shared decision-making process, when appropriate.
- Aim to establish a diverse healthful practice/work environment at all levels, including leadership and governance teams.
- Celebrate the diversity of talent as a source of strength, pride, and team spirit throughout the organization.
- Emphasize the promotion, recognition, and acceptance of diversity by all staff members in a non-biased and sensitive manner.
- Facilitate the creation of a work environment that is conducive to open communication, flexibility, and acceptance of differences.
- Lead staff members without stereotypes or assumptions and with sensitivity to their gender, race/ethnicity, knowledge, skills, cultural backgrounds, values, and beliefs.
- Establish metrics to monitor targeted diversity benchmarks.

Guiding principle 3: Health care organizations will partner with universities, schools of nursing, and other organizations that train health care workers to support development and implementation of policies, procedures, programs, and learning environments that foster recruitment and retention of a student population that reflects the diversity of the United States

- Encourage use of admission criteria that focus on both qualitative and quantitative data.
- Recognize and appreciate the social and cultural barriers to college attendance that may exist for students from diverse population groups.
- Enter into collaborative agreements between education and practice that offer nursing staff from diverse groups the opportunity to serve as student mentors, guest lecturers, participants in school-based health centers, and/or clinical faculty.
- Encourage and support graduate education for nurses from diverse populations to build a more diverse pool of nurse leaders including nursing faculty.
- Develop and implement career plans for potential candidates for nursing careers from current employees with an emphasis on those from non-majority groups.
- Create and support community outreach programs such as shadow a nurse day, health care career fairs, and high school tutoring programs for targeted cultural groups in collaboration with members of the local community.

- Create a clinical rotation environment that supports a diverse nursing student body and learning styles.

Guiding principle 4: Health care organizations will collect and disseminate diversity related resources and information

- Use technology to heighten awareness and share information and resources related to diversity.
- Collect data (including, but not limited to, race and primary language spoken) as a part of routine patient registration processes and human resources management programs to better document and reflect the components of the patient and workforce populations. Establish formal policies and procedures to reflect these data collections.
- Support health care information technology (IT) systems that enhance the collection of diverse patient and workforce demographic data.
- Provide education to all staff regarding the relevance and value of collecting patient and workforce data including race, ethnicity and primary language spoken. Train staff on effective strategies and appropriate mechanisms for obtaining these data elements.
- Inform communities why it is necessary for health care organizations to collect patient and workforce race, ethnicity and primary language data.
- Routinely review quality and use data by race, ethnicity and primary language of patients to eliminate potential inconsistency in quality of care across various patient populations and to balance patient population demographics and the workforce population.
- Use data to develop action plans toward improving the state of diversity in the workplace.
- Conduct research to measure the effectiveness of improvement plans.
- Review evidence-based practice, related to diversity, and incorporate "best practices" into the organizations' own settings.

From the American Organization of Nurse Executives (AONE). Available at: www.aone.org. Accessed May 28, 2008; with permission.

---

perspectives about the disease that enable people to make sense of their experience. People with chronic illness live in "the dual kingdoms of the well and the sick" bouncing back and forth. The major factors identified as fostering exchange of prominences in the foreground is the perception of a threat to control and the recognition that the shift or bounce has occurred and a need to return to the closest state of wellness possible.[28] The measure of wellness is determined by comparing the experience with what is known and understood about illness and vice versa. According to the shifting perspectives model, the perspectives are not right or wrong but rather "reflect people's needs and situations." The basis of the model is also true in today's rapidly changing demographic

interactions. It is even more so for individuals who are not of the majority. The many frameworks are in a way the shifting perspectives as captured by the model's developer. Applying this model to the cultural competency dilemma as an overarching framework shows promise as a way of conceptualizing the concepts, constructs, and relationships that form the complex and dynamic realm of culturally congruent health care and furthers the understanding of the many cultural competence frameworks in general.

Schematically, the shifting perspectives model looks like an eclipse where the majority culture is the sun and difference is the moon. Each perspective is depicted by overlapping circles in which either the majority culture or difference takes precedence. As the reality of the individual's experience and the personal and social context changes, the individual's perspectives shift in the degree to which difference is in the foreground or background of their "world." Past experiences also play a role in when difference shifts into the foreground for an individual. A person's past experiences, such as confronting racism, are always lurking in the shadows and can be pulled to the forefront based on the situation faced. Ignoring past experiences does not erase them or the residual effects they leave.

The perception of reality, not the reality itself, is the essence of how people interpret and respond

---

Box 2
The purpose of MODELS

Makes sense of the relationships of the parts

Opens the mindset of the user

Develops individuals and organizations

Eliminates barriers to the desired outcome

Leads the user in the direction of the preferred state

Self-examination through questioning; ask questions…then ask more questions to their experiences. One's perspectives form and shape their realities. Gone are the days of failing to consider or outright ignoring the views, feelings, and interpretations of others. Multiple realities can and do inhabit the same space simultaneously. Because this country believes in individual rights, it is expected and extolled that personal reality receives consideration and respect. The sheer existence of these multiple perspectives is at the heart of the complexities and challenges of cultural competence. All of the cultural competence frameworks capture this phenomenon. Considering and using the knowledge and mandates of the patient's culture provides the ability to operationalize culturally competent care within the nursing process. To do so requires learning the "how tos," which includes asking questions, holding in abeyance assumptions and ethnocentricism, and learning more about different worldviews and that which is unfamiliar and sometimes taboo. Each emphasizes the need to learn about one's self and about other cultures, a proposition that is nonending and requires continuous learning.

SUMMARY

Culture: individuals possess it, organizations have it too, countries flaunt it with pride, professions and religious denominations are forms of it. Because every customer encounter (whether patient or a coworker) is a cultural encounter, using creative ways to approach content of this nature is always welcomed. Culture is the lens through which the world is viewed and approached. It influences decisions made, actions taken, and personal relations. One cannot operate for any length of time in a way that is inconsistent with one's own thinking. Culture is everywhere and exists in a variety of forms that often collide with each other, creating at times horrendous moments and at others quite humorous, but always instructional occasions. Because all knowledge is about the past and all decisions are about the future, mental models suggest that the quest to be the best requires continuous learning. When one puts culture and competence together (cultural competence), the result is both a process (series of events) and an outcome (a synthesis of different perspectives). Mastering the skill set of cultural competence is a win-win for all involved. In health care, this understanding is what is needed for the demands of today's unique patient and workforce.

REFERENCES

1. King ML. At the second national convention of the medical committee for human rights. In: Satcher D, Pamies RJ, editors. Multicultural Medicine and Health Disparities. Columbus (OH): The McGraw-Hill Companies, Inc.; 2006. p. 405.
2. American Organization of Nurse Executives position statement and guiding principles for diversity in health care organizations. Available at: http://www.aone.org. Accessed May 28, 2008.
3. Gruman JC. An expanded view of health: implications for how healthcare works. Behav Med 1994; 20:119–22.
4. US Department of Health and Human Services' Office of Minority Health (USDHH OMH). Final report: national standards for culturally and linguistically appropriate services in health care. Washington, DC: OCR; 2001.
5. Division of Standards and Survey Methods. Joint Commission standards supporting the provision of culturally and linguistically appropriate standards. Oakbrook Terrace (IL): Author; 2007.
6. Sullivan Commission on Diversity in the Healthcare Workforce. Missing persons: minorities in the health professions. Washington, DC: Sullivan Commission; 2004.
7. Institute of Medicine. Committee on understanding and eliminating racial and ethnic disparities in health care, board on health sciences policy. Unequal treatment: confronting racial and ethnic disparities in healthcare. Washington, DC: The National Academies Press; 2002.
8. Thomas DA. The truth about mentoring minorities: race matters. Harvard Business Review Product 2179; 2002. p. 55–63.
9. Hall ET. The silent language. Garden City, New York: Doubleday and Company; 1959.
10. Hernandez M, Hodges S. Crafting logic models for systems of care: ideas into action. [Making children's mental health services successful series, volume 1]. Tampa, FL: University of South Florida, The Louis de la Parte Florida Mental Health Institute, Department of Child & Family Studies; 2003.
11. Hernandez M, Hodges S. Theory-based accountability. In: Hernandez M, Hodges PH, editors. Developing outcome strategies in children's mental health. Baltimore (MD): Brookes Publishing Co; 2001. p. 21–40.
12. Edge R. One middle-age white male's perspective on racism and cultural competence: a view from the bunker where we wait to have our privilege stripped away. Ment Retard 2002;40(1):83–5.
13. US Department of Health and Human Services' Office of Minority Health (USDHH OMH). Teaching cultural competence in health care: a review of current concepts, policies and practices. Contract Number: 282-98-0029, Task Order #41. March 12, 2002.
14. Jirwe M, Gerrish K, Emami A. The Theoretical framework of cultural competence. Journal of Multicultural Nursing & Health 2006;12(3):6–16.

15. Andrews MM, Boyle JS. Transcultural concepts in nursing care. 4th edition. Philadelphia: Lippincott Williams & Wilkins; 2003.
16. Campinha-Bacote J. The process of cultural competence in the delivery of healthcare services: a culturally competent model of care. 4th edition. Cincinnati (OH): Transcultural C.A.R.E. Associates; 2003.
17. Giger JN, Davidizhar RE. Transcultural nursing: assessment & intervention. 4th edition. St. Louis (MO): Mosby; 2004.
18. Leininger M, McFarland MR. Transcultural nursing: concepts, theories, research and practice. 3rd edition. New York: McGraw-Hill; 2002.
19. Lipson JG, Steiger NJ. Self-care nursing in a multicultural context. Thousand Oaks, CA; London: Sage; 1996.
20. Papadopoulos I, Tilki M, Taylor G. Transcultural care: a guide for health care professionals. Dinton (UK): Quay Books; 1998.
21. Purnell LD, Paulanka BJ. Transcultural healthcare: a culturally competent approach. Philadelphia: F.A. Davis; 2003.
22. Spector RE. Cultural diversity in health and illness. 6th edition. Upper Saddle River (NJ): Prentice Hall; 2004.
23. Wepa D, editor. Cultural safety in Aotearoa, New Zealand. Auckland (New Zealand): Pearson Education; 2005. p. 6–16.
24. Schim S, Doorenbos A, Benkert R, et al. Culturally congruent care: putting the puzzle together. J Transcult Nurs 2007;18(2):103–10.
25. Camphina-Bacote J. A biblically based model of cultural competence in healthcare delivery. Journal of Multicultural Nursing & Health 2005;11(2):16–22.
26. Kim-Goodwin YS, Clarke PN, Barton L. A model for the delivery of culturally competent community care. J Adv Nurs 2001;35(6):918–25.
27. Sofaer S, Firminger K. Patient perceptions of the quality of health services. Annu Rev Public Health 2005;26:513–59.
28. Paterson BL. The shifting perspectives model of chronic illness. J Nurs Scholarsh 2001;33(1):21–32.

A Collaborative Curricular Model for Implementing Evidence-Based Nursing in a Critical Care Setting

Kathryn M. Ewers, RN, BA, MEd[a,b,]*,
Carol T. Coker, ARNP, MSN, CWOCN[c],
Irmajean Bajnok, RN, MScN, PhD[d], Ann Lynn Denker, ARNP, PhD[b,e,f]

KEYWORDS

- Collaboration • Curricular model
- Evidence-based nursing practice • Champion building

As more and more hospitals embark on the magnet journey, strategies for providing evidence-based practice (EBP) as a standard for nursing excellence become paramount. The American Nurses Association[1] and the American Nurses Credentialing Center,[2] a subsidiary of the American Nurses Association, recognize EBP standards as critical to providing excellent nursing care. The American Nurses Credentialing Center Magnet Recognition Program[3] is a prestigious recognition of nursing services in health care organizations.

Magnet hospital designation is based on meeting standards for 14 Forces of Magnetism. EBP standards emanate primarily from Magnet Force 6, Quality of Care. To meet the standards of this force, institutions must be able to show that research and EBPs are embedded into both clinical and operational practices. Institutions must also show evidence of high-quality research and

evidenced-based care to patients and families. Research studies[4–7] show that Magnet-designated hospitals enjoy benefits not only relating to improvements in nursing care quality, but also to lowering mortality rates, increasing patient satisfaction, and enhancing nurse recruitment and retention.

As part of the quality component of the magnet recognition program, health care organizations must monitor nurse and patient satisfaction and patient falls, pressure ulcer rates, and other nurse-sensitive quality indicators.[2] The National Database of Nursing Quality Indicators (NDNQI) is a national nursing quality measurement program that provides health care organizations with unit-level performance reports and comparisons with national averages, percentile rankings, and other data services.[2] **Table 1** illustrates the NDNQI indicators[8] and those measures endorsed by the National Quality Forum[9] that are part of the

[a] Education and Development, Jackson Health System, 1500 NW 12th Avenue, 7th Floor East Towers, Miami, FL 33136, USA
[b] University of Miami School of Nursing and Health Studies, Coral Gables, FL, USA
[c] Jackson Health System, 1611 NW 12th Avenue, Wound Ostomy Continence Management, Park Plaza Room 301B, Miami, FL 33136, USA
[d] Registered Nurses' Association of Ontario, 158 Pearl Street, Toronto, Ontario, Canada M5H 1L3
[e] Jackson Health System, 1611 NW 12th Avenue, Miami, FL 33136, USA
[f] Center for Nursing Excellence, Jackson Medical Towers, 1500 NW 12th Avenue, 7th Floor East Towers, Room 709C, Miami, FL 33136, USA
* Corresponding author. Education and Development, Jackson Health System, 1500 NW 12th Avenue, 7th Floor East Towers, Miami, FL 33136.
E-mail address: kewers@jhsmiami.org (K.M. Ewers).

Crit Care Nurs Clin N Am 20 (2008) 423–434
doi:10.1016/j.ccell.2008.08.007

Table 1
National Database of Nursing Quality Indicators

Indicator	Subindicator
Patient falls[a]	
Patient falls with injury[a]	
Pressure ulcers	Community
	Hospital acquired
	Unit acquired
Staff mix[a]	
Nursing hours per patient day[a]	
Registered nurse surveys	Job satisfaction
	Practice environment scale[a]
Registered nurse education and certification	
Pediatric pain assessment cycle	
Pediatric IV infiltration rate	
Psychiatric patient assault rate	
Restraints prevalence[a]	
Nurse turnover[a]	
Nosocomial infections	Ventilator-assisted pneumonia[a]
	Central line–associated bloodstream infection[a]
	Catheter-associated urinary tract infections[a]

[a] Key indicators are also part of the National Quality Forum's Nursing Sensitive Measure Set.

National Quality Forum Nursing Sensitive Measure Set. Institutional participation in this database facilitates nursing and organizational knowledge of the quality of their care and provides a systematic process that measures and analyzes outcomes to drive nursing quality improvement initiatives.

As Jackson Health System (JHS), one of the largest public, academic affiliated hospitals in the United States, embarked on the magnet journey, the nursing quality indicator of pressure ulcer prevalence was monitored by the NDNQI database. This article describes how the partnership with the Registered Nurses' Association of Ontario (RNAO) and the subsequent implementation of the RNAO's nursing best practice guideline (BPG) Risk Assessment and Prevention of Pressure Ulcers[10] in the critical care areas evolved to become an important component of an evidence-based nursing collaborative curriculum. Institutions grappling with how to meet EBP standards required for designation as a Magnet hospital may find this case study instructive.

THE DYNAMICS OF EMBARKING ON AN INTERNATIONAL PARTNERSHIP WITH THE REGISTERED NURSES' ASSOCIATION OF ONTARIO

The development of an international partnership between JHS and RNAO and the endorsement of practice guidelines as a viable strategy for implementing evidence-based nursing care evolved over a 2-year period. To understand how JHS aligned the RNAO guidelines with the Magnet journey, a brief overview of both American and Canadian contexts of guideline implementation is helpful.

American and Canadian Guideline Implementation Contexts

In the United States, nursing specialty groups, such as the Wound Ostomy Continence Society, or hospital-affiliated academic centers are leading nursing guideline development and dissemination. Despite the endorsement by the Agency for Healthcare Research and Quality to use clinical practice guidelines as a key strategy for implementing EBP, only 5% of the total guidelines available from the United States repository for clinical practice guidelines, the National Guideline Clearinghouse, are nursing guidelines. Of the 106 nursing guidelines found on this site,[11] approximately 30% are foreign, with Canada, through RNAO, contributing most of the foreign guidelines.[11] A recent national nursing research study evaluating the readiness of American nurses for EBP[12] and an EBP study from an international organization[13] neglected to survey participants about practice guideline use as a relevant source of "best evidence" or as a credible resource for research use. Conclusions from these respective studies were that nurses were not ready for EBP and that appraisal and analysis were the most challenging aspects of the EBP process.[12,13]

In contrast to the United States context, Canadian nurse leaders and organizations although not engaging in the Magnet journey, endorsed evidence-based nursing practice standards and clinical practice guideline adoption in the late 1990s. In 1999, RNAO received multiyear funding from the Ontario Ministry of Health and Long Term Care to launch the Nursing Best Practice Guideline Program. This program supports the provision of point-of-care evidence-based nursing practice by way of guideline development, dissemination, and implementation. In 2000, Judith Shamian, Executive Director of the Office of Nursing Policy, Health Canada, proclaimed the development of BPGs as the most important nursing project of the generation.[14] By 2008, RNAO had developed 31 clinical practice guidelines and six healthy work environment BPGs, had led the implementation of these guidelines in over 47 health care institutions in Ontario, and had become recognized as a world leader in nursing guideline development and implementation.[15] Canadian health care institutions that commit to implementation, evaluation, and dissemination of RNAO BPGs can be designated as Best Practice Spotlight Organizations.[16] Attainment of this status is recognition of the institution's commitment to delivery of excellent nursing care through implementation of BPGs.

Canadian nurses use practice guidelines as a tool to facilitate the EBP process. JHS used the RNAO guidelines as a key strategy for meeting EBP standards required for Magnet hospital designation.

Timeline and Dynamics of Becoming the First International Registered Nurses' Association of Ontario Center Member

As early as the late 1990s, the clinical Wound Ostomy Continence Nurse (WOCN) expert at JHS was already using guidelines from the Wound Ostomy Continence Society and the Agency for Healthcare Policy and Research as a basis for evidence-based pressure ulcer care. There was no nursing strategy or plan, however, to implement practice guidelines in a systematic way. In 2003, 3 years before the development of an international partnership between JHS and RNAO and the endorsement of practice guidelines as a viable strategy for meeting EBP standards required for Magnet Hospital designation, a Canadian nurse educator working at JHS had informally introduced BPGs into several continuing education classes. Working collaboratively with the hospital's WOCN clinical expert and with members of the WOCN team, RNAO's guidelines and World Wide Web–based resources related to pressure ulcer prevention and care were evaluated. The team evaluated the RNAO guidelines and found these to be synonymous with the American Wound Ostomy Continence Society and Agency for Healthcare Policy and Research guidelines already in use. Major advantages of the RNAO's guidelines were that the guidelines included practice, education, and policy recommendations; had accompanying implementation resources, such as the Toolkit: Implementation of Clinical Practice Guidelines;[17] were World Wide Web accessible; and were in the public domain. Guidelines and accompanying resources could be easily downloaded and copied without copyright infringement. These guidelines were easily accessible at no cost to practitioners at the point of care.

When the hospital formally initiated the Magnet Journey, an educational strategic plan for EBP was developed. Armed with the knowledge that RNAO had been helping Canadian nurses implement EBP using guideline implementation since 1999, the plan was presented to senior nursing leadership. In June 2004, senior leadership at JHS supported an educator to attend the weeklong residential RNAO summer institute on Best Practice Guidelines in Ontario, Canada, hosted by the RNAO Center for Professional Nursing Excellence, to advance the development of an educational strategic plan. By January 2005, a hospital-based Certificate in Evidence-Based Nursing was developed at JHS. Integral to this four-course certificate program was curriculum content on guideline implementation. This content was introduced to all new nurses in orientation sessions at hospital-wide continuing education classes. Clinical nurse educators and policy and procedure committee members were also targeted for introduction to guidelines as key strategy for providing evidence-based care.

In June 2005, an online EBP survey was developed to acquire a baseline benchmark regarding JHS nurses' knowledge of EBP. Results of the survey indicated that although 46% of the nurses did have knowledge about the existence of practice guidelines, only 3.5% used guidelines to answer clinical questions.[18] Clearly, educational initiatives in addition to the Certificate in Evidence-Based Nursing needed to occur for nurses to embrace guideline implementation.

EBP survey data were shared with the RNAO and the idea of creating a Best Practice Champions Network and developing evidence-based champions to implement guidelines was proposed. To operationalize this, RNAO recommended JHS become a member of the RNAO Center. The RNAO Center is the professional development arm of RNAO that provides education and consultation services to health care organizations who purchase membership to enhance nursing excellence and quality patient care. By year's end, JHS became the first international RNAO Center member. This membership entitled the JHS to consultation and facilitation services related to an individualized action plan focused on implementing selected BPGs.

In January 2006, senior nursing leadership at JHS contracted the help of an external consultant to advance Magnet planning. As a result, a nursing vision and a strategic plan were developed that supported the implementation of EBP. Practice guideline implementation was identified as a strategy for demonstrating EBP. Leadership selected pressure ulcer prevention in the critical care areas as the most urgent clinical problem that guideline implementation should address. This assessment was made in response to compelling historical JHS pressure ulcer prevalence scores, the need to meet Magnet practice standards, and knowledge of potential legislative reimbursement changes for pressure ulcer care by the Centers for Medicare and Medicaid. Funding for RNAO Center membership was secured and from May to October a series of evidence-based skin champion and leadership workshops was held.

Strategies for Organizational Impact and Sustainability

Initial strategies for organizational impact and sustainability included a multistep process. First, a 2-day workshop on leading and sustaining change for nursing leaders was conducted. Second, a 1-day champion-building workshop for clinical educators working in noncritical care areas was held. Third, policies and procedures were reviewed to make sure they were aligned with the RNAO guideline recommendations. Lastly, integration of guideline recommendations into medical, surgical, and critical nursing internships, orientation sessions, and continuing education classes was facilitated. As shared governance structures took hold across the organization, unit practice councils increasingly became a more effective way to lead the practice changes recommended in the RNAO guidelines.

ESTABLISHING AN EVIDENCE-BASED CURRICULUM FRAMEWORK AND METHODOLOGY
Overview

A key role of the RNAO Center for Professional Nursing Excellence in the partnership with JHS was to lead the planning, development, and delivery of a relevant professional development program to facilitate quality evidence-based nursing care. This involved developing a program for skin care champions selected from the leaders of the critical care units involved in this initiative. The program focused on the role of EBP champion; knowledge about EBP and implementing BPGs; and specific information related to assessment, prevention, and management of pressure ulcers. The program development work also involved establishing a second series of workshops on leading and sustaining change for managers, directors, and educators.

Program Development Process for Champions

The program development process was initiated with the JHS team and members of the RNAO Center and RNAO BPGs experts. Through a series of teleconference sessions, the goals, themes, and specific areas of focus were established for all the workshops. The overall curricular framework reflected an approach that began with the practitioner and the role each was expected to play as critical care skin champions. From there, the focus was on expansion of the champions' knowledge base related to EBP, BPGs, and how best practices are most successfully implemented. The RNAO BPG Implementation Toolkit[17] was used as a guide to assist participants to select, assess, implement, and evaluate guideline use. Following this component of the curriculum, the participants had an understanding of the role of a champion, and considerable background knowledge related to BPGs. The skin champions were now ready to learn the details of the specific guideline focused on risk assessment and prevention of pressure ulcers.[19] **Fig. 1** outlines the key content areas of focus in the inaugural workshops.[20] **Fig. 2** further describes the curricular model.[21]

It was important in the curricular design to make sure that at the outset the participants knew what was expected of them in their role as champions. This meant that they viewed all further content through the lens of being a champion. All workshop sessions consisted of content presented in concise integrated segments introducing theory and providing participants with the opportunity to reflect on how the

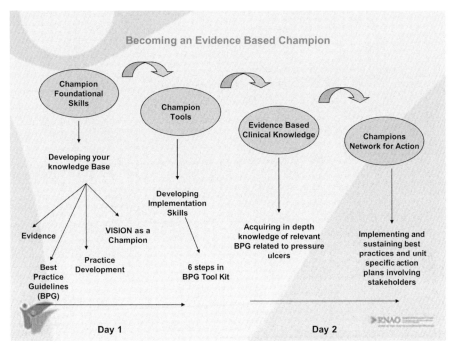

Fig. 1. Key content areas for champions' workshop. (*Courtesy of* Registered Nurses Association of Ontario, Toronto, Ontario, Canada.)

information was related to their practice and their role as clinical leaders and champions. For each knowledge segment, participants were involved in a practical application activity to facilitate the new knowledge in a meaningful way. The sessions involved considerable group work, given that guideline implementation generally occurs best in unit-based teams who plan and develop strategies they agree to carry out together.[22] This teaching methodology was selected because the participants were practitioners accustomed to physically active days, were interested in gaining knowledge that would influence their day-to-day practice, and often worked in teams to deliver nursing care.

Participants were exceptionally engaged, embracing the opportunities to hear how they could best use the content in practice. From the outset, the participants were placed in small groups to work together as a team, mirroring how they might work in implementation teams with their staff. After the planned "getting acquainted" sessions, each small group developed a team identity, theme, and vision that they used throughout the workshops. Beginning with the first exercise, small groups were expected to learn how to report processes and outcomes and share their work both creatively and concisely.

Program Development Process for Managers and Directors

The second component of this professional development program enhanced the knowledge of managers and directors throughout JHS. The goals were to build support for the work of champions in the critical care units and to promote spread of the evidence-based culture; the champion model (see **Fig. 1**);[21] and use of the RNAO Implementation Tool Kit.[22] Recognizing that change must be both bottom up and top down for it to succeed, the JHS leadership complemented the unit-based approaches reinforced through the critical care skin champion workshops. Through discussion with various JHS personnel and with members of the RNAO Center and healthy work environment experts, a curriculum focused on leadership and change was developed. Leadership support is recognized as a component of a healthy work environment and is closely linked with the uptake and sustained use of clinical best practices.[23,24]

The curricular model of leading and sustaining change used both the RNAO Healthy Work Environment Best Practice Guideline: Developing and Sustaining Nursing Leadership[25] and Bridges'[26] work related to transitions. It is particularly important to acknowledge the concept of "transitions" when focusing on a major cultural change. This

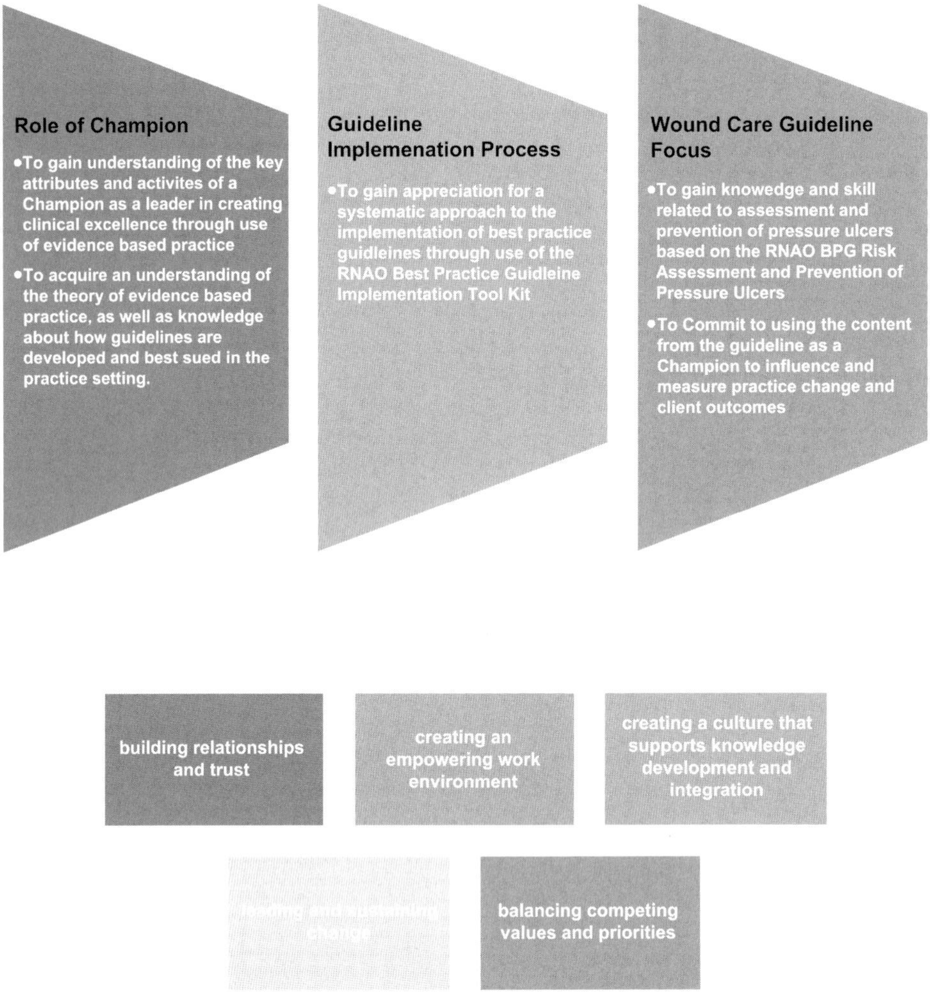

Role of Champion

● To gain understanding of the key attributes and activites of a Champion as a leader in creating clinical excellence through use of evidence based practice

● To acquire an understanding of the theory of evidence based practice, as well as knowledge about how guidelines are developed and best sued in the practice setting.

Guideline Implemenation Process

● To gain appreciation for a systematic approach to the implementation of best practice guidleines through use of the RNAO Best Practice Guideleine Implementation Tool Kit

Wound Care Guideline Focus

● To gain knowedge and skill related to assessment and prevention of pressure ulcers based on the RNAO BPG Risk Assessment and Prevention of Pressure Ulcers

● To Commit to using the content from the guideline as a Champion to influence and measure practice change and client outcomes

building relationships and trust

creating an empowering work environment

creating a culture that supports knowledge development and integration

leading and sustaining change

balancing competing values and priorities

Fig. 2. Curricular model for critical care skin champions.

understanding enables identification of current strengths, areas that must be given up, and new practices that will be adopted. If the transition from one state to another is effectively managed through a successful change process, resistance can be greatly reduced and all members of the team can be supported to feel they have a contribution to make. If such an approach is not used, long-time staff may feel that as their practices are changing, they themselves may be perceived as obsolete and may tend to resist changes to the status quo. This work on transitions was augmented by a focus on the leadership model included in the RNAO leadership guideline.[25] The five transformational leadership practices of (1) building relationships and trust, (2) creating an empowering work environment, (3) creating a culture that supports knowledge development and integration, (4) leading and sustaining change, and (5) balancing competing values and priorities,

were emphasized. **Fig. 3** further identifies the relationship between the five transformational leadership practices, organizational supports, personal resources, and outcomes.[25]

Planning and Implementation Challenges

The development and conduction of 6 days of workshops from a distance involving two different countries and two different health care systems had its challenges. The challenges were balanced by the fact that the two organizations, RNAO and JHS, had congruent values related to nurses as knowledge professionals, quality care, and excellence in nursing practice.

The standard challenges of never enough time, cultural differences in health care systems between Canada and the United States, the realities of working with practitioners who can never be totally relieved of their patient care responsibilities

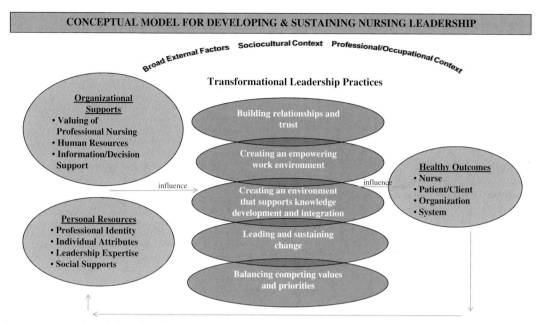

Fig. 3. Conceptual model for developing and sustaining leadership. (*Courtesy of* Registered Nurses Association of Ontario, Toronto, Ontario, Canada.)

to engage in a workshop, and such issues as sustaining the motivation between workshops were all evident. To overcome these challenges, the workshops provided opportunities for participants to give feedback throughout and at the end of each session, which led to modifications that enhanced subsequent workshops. Participants were also encouraged to spend time on applying the workshop content to their own contexts and to focus on specific plans and next steps. These activities helped participants sustain the momentum for implementing practice changes, between and after all the sessions.

In general, the challenges were minimized because both organizations embraced EBP. Both organizations believed in using multiple approaches to achieve clinical excellence. Both organizations believed that champions and leaders were critical in implementing and sustaining practice changes based on BPGs. Lastly, both organizations were committed to a successful partnership that would influence an evidence-based nursing culture, and positive patient outcomes.

PARTNERSHIP OUTCOMES
Practice Outcomes

Historically, pressure ulcer data collection at JHS had been conducted on an annual and biannual basis. From as early as 1999, JHS collected data by internal prevalence and incidence surveys benchmarking data against multiple national and

international sources. Despite these efforts, prevalence rates remained unacceptably above the reported national and international benchmarks, including those of NDNQI. Pressure ulcer data results were not addressed systematically across the organization. In 2005, data collection for NDNQI revealed that the prevalence of hospital-acquired pressure ulcers was greater than twice the national benchmarked mean. Recently, the Centers for Medicare and Medicaid services have listed pressure ulcer development as a "never event" and do not reimburse for related care at institutions where patients develop greater than stage one pressure ulcers.[27]

The RNAO skin champion workshops in tandem with the organizational push to meet Magnet EBP standards served as powerful catalysts for practice changes. Overall, the champion workshops and subsequent implementation of the BPG Risk Assessment and Prevention of Pressure Ulcers[19] resulted in four major outcomes: (1) dramatic initial decrease in pressure ulcer prevalence, (2) heightened awareness of the importance and value of low-technology evidence-based skin care practices for the critically ill patient, (3) development and implementation of evidence-based skin care–related practice innovations, and (4) identification of strategies for sustaining practice changes. **Table 2** highlights the general components of the summary of recommendations participants consulted to make practice changes.[28] Specific practice recommendations for each

Table 2
Components of the Registered Nurses' Association of Ontario best practice guidelines summary: risk assessment and prevention of pressure ulcers

Component	Subcomponent
Practice recommendations	Assessment
	Planning
	Interventions
	Discharge, transfer of care arrangements
Education recommendations	
Organization and policy recommendations	
Levels of evidence associated with each recommendation	

component of the guideline are identified as part of the summary of recommendations.

RNAO practice recommendations regarding interventions for individuals restricted to bed were particularly relevant to the critical care skin champions. As unit-based champions implemented intensive evidence-based pressure ulcer prevention practices, unit-acquired pressure ulcer prevalence dramatically declined to within NDNQI prevalence rates. Champions became more aware of their "ICU mindset" that typically valued the care priorities of high technology skills (monitoring of ventilator status, and administration of critical intravenous medications) over what was viewed as less life-saving, low technology skin care interventions. Confronting the attitude that "after all, a patient can live with a pressure ulcer" was pivotal to helping nurses initiate and sustain practice changes.

Unit champions developed and implemented several skin care innovations. Examples of these included development of a standardized data pressure ulcer prevalence collection tool, "hotlisting" patients at high risk for pressure ulcer development, and implementation of team huddles to focus attention on specific pressure ulcer prevention and risk reduction interventions. Champions also shared pressure ulcer data by way of bulletin boards, unit-based newsletters, staff meetings, and interdisciplinary groups. However, as competing corporate initiatives emerged, pressure ulcer prevalence began to increase even in units that had been most successful in reducing pressure ulcer prevalence. In response to this, a Critical Care Pressure Ulcer Task Force (CCPUTF) was established. The task force led by the WOCN coordinator and the Critical Care Assistant Director of Nursing established weekly 1-hour sessions where open dialog was shared among the nurse managers and educators. Unit-based champions

contributed to the dialog by identifying and addressing barriers to practice change. The CCPUTF became a supportive format where both leadership and nurses could share best practices and discuss barriers to evidence-based skin care practices.

Members of the CCPUTF noted that units that enjoyed high unit leadership engagement also were more likely to sustain practice changes. This insight is consistent with recent research[24] linking high leadership engagement with sustainability of practice change over time. The CCPUTF has played an important role in keeping ulcer pressure prevention at the forefront in the critical care setting and in returning the pressure ulcer prevalence to within NDNQI rates.

Educational and Organizational Outcomes

Over 100 skin care champions and nearly 100 nursing leaders attended the leading and sustaining change workshops in 2006. Within the first year postguideline implementation, members of the critical care skin champion network had sponsored a successful interdisciplinary pressure ulcer prevention educational fair, developed an educational skin care newsletter, and continued to present their insights into guideline implementation at a variety of national and international conferences.

A postguideline implementation survey comparing JHS nurses with Canadian nurses using the Perceived Worth of Best Practice Guidelines Scale and the Educational and Supported Processes Scale[29] was completed. The survey data showed that like the Canadian nurses, JHS nurses found BPGs useful and valuable for implementing evidence-based nursing practices changes. Similarly, JHS nurses agreed that the educational and supportive processes were adequate. When asked about the likelihood of consulting other

BPGs to address other clinical questions, respondents overwhelmingly indicated they would consult other guidelines.

Unit practice councils began to take the lead in using guidelines to provide more EBP changes. With over 100 practice councils under development institution-wide, the potential of EBP changes was immense. Examples of RNAO clinical and healthy work environment BPGs that councils and task forces have embraced include Assessment and Device Selection and Maintenance to Reduce Vascular Access Complication,[30,31] Prevention of Falls and Fall Injuries in the Older Adult,[32] Women Abuse: Screening, Identification and Initial Response,[33] Embracing Cultural Diversity in Healthcare: Developing Cultural Competence,[34] and Collaborative Practice Among Nursing Teams Guideline.[35] Additionally in 2006, five nurses showed their interest in guideline implementation by volunteering to become stakeholder reviewers for RNAO healthy work environment guidelines then under development. Subsequently, a 2008 call by RNAO for stakeholder reviewers for additional guidelines being developed generated more interest and participation by JHS nurses.

Guideline implementation and the partnership with RNAO also helped to foster broader interest in research and EBP. Senior nursing leadership at JHS collaborated with research faculty from the University of Miami School of Nursing and Health Studies to fund an onsite Certificate in Nursing Research for interested JHS nurses and nurses from the community. In 2007, six JHS nurses graduated with a Certificate in Nursing Research. A JHS hospital nurse educator who held adjunct faculty status at the University of Miami School of Nursing and Health Studies lectured on guideline implementation as part of the nursing curricula for the Nursing Research Certificate and the Certificate in Nursing Education. This is an example of how educators in a practice setting can help reduce the learning gap between theory, research, and practice.

The most ambitious outcome stemming from the initial partnership with RNAO was the renewal of RNAO Center membership in 2007 with the commitment to plan a collaborative South Florida Winter Evidence-Based Nursing Institute and an Evidence-Based Nursing Conference: Bringing Best Evidence to the Point of Care. These events were held in January 2008. Over 75 JHS nurses were funded to attend these EBP events. Fourteen JHS nurses and several other American and Canadian nurses showcased their EBP projects at these exciting inaugural events. To kick off the research conference, a gala reception was held where RNAO's healthy work environment best practice guideline[36] on staffing and workload was unveiled to local politicians, the Canadian Consul, hospital

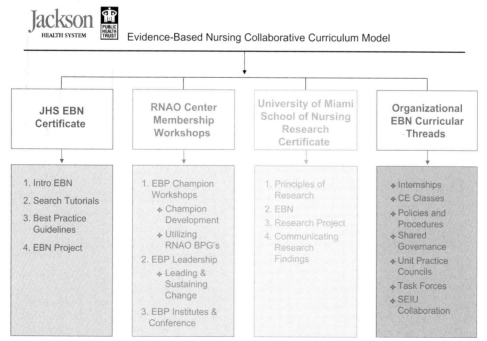

Fig. 4. Evidence-based nursing collaborative curriculum model. (*Courtesy of* Jackson Health System, Miami, Florida.)

board members, and the academic and nursing community at large. The event served to highlight the staffing and workload guideline and the importance of effective staffing and workload for nurses based on the strong growing evidence relating patient care outcomes to the number and type of nursing staff. Overall, the events provided nurses with many opportunities for cross-cultural sharing of nursing knowledge and clinical practices setting the stage for future collaborations.

Participant evaluations of these EBP events resoundingly proclaimed the value of the international partnership. Nurses overwhelmingly commented that they found the presentations to be informative and inspirational. This speaks not only to the quality of the presentations, but also to the value of providing and supporting clinical staff development as a cornerstone for changing professional practices. The collaborative nature of the project provided unprecedented opportunity for nurses in all sectors and roles publicly to support and demonstrate the collective goal of providing evidence-based quality nursing care.

Not only were clinical staff nurses and practice council members revitalized by these EBP events, but also these events helped raise the consciousness of senior leadership to nursings' accomplishments at JHS. Many of the partnership outcomes were presented to senior leadership at the Shared Governance Council meeting. These outcomes were used as part of the research and EBP annual report. Data from this report helped nursing leaders identify funding and budget recommendations for future research and EBP events. All of these outcomes provided strong evidence to support the EBP standards of Magnet Force 6. In addition, JHS has been invited to submit a proposal to RNAO to be the first International Best Practice Spotlight Organization[16] based on their organization-wide leading-edge guideline implementation and evaluation work in the United States.

SUMMARY

The JHS partnership with RNAO is an outstanding example of the importance of international collaboration for identifying viable strategies, curricular models, and resources for implementing EBP standards. Guideline implementation may be an excellent strategy for implementing EBP standards and a helpful tool for institutions on the Magnet journey. As such, curricular models need to include guideline implementation as part of the overall EBP curriculum. BPG champion network workshops and subsequent evidence-based nursing institutes are valuable methods for introducing nurses to evidence-based nursing practices and guideline implementation. **Fig. 4** illustrates how guideline implementation is integrated into the JHS evidence-based nursing curriculum model and could be a framework useful to other organizations.[37]

Finally, more nursing research is needed to evaluate the effectiveness of guideline implementation as a valuable research tool. The case study described throughout this article illustrates that the use of meaningful resources, such as evidence-based guidelines, implementation tools, and creative educational programming tailored to the personal and organizational context, can be powerful facilitators of research use in nursing practice. Recent nursing research[38] suggests that predictors of research use include hospital size, time spent on the Internet, level of nurse exhaustion, quality of facilitation, nurse-to-nurse collaboration, the nature of the nursing culture, and perceptions of the ability to control practice. Accordingly, nurse leaders who wish to foster EBPs need to consider the complexities of research use and guideline implementation.

ACKNOWLEDGMENTS

The authors thank Jane Mass, Senior VP of Nursing, Jackson Health System, and the faculty of the Center for Nursing Excellence at Jackson Health System, for their outstanding support of international RNAO Center Membership as a key strategy for implementing evidence-based nursing practice. They also wish to thank Martha Baker, RN, Nurse Manager of Trauma ICU, Jackson Health System, and President of Service Employees International Union, Local 1991, and the faculty of the University of Miami School of Nursing and Health Studies for supporting evidence-based nursing practice events.

REFERENCES

1. American Nurses Association (ANA). Nursing: scope and standards of practice. Washington, DC: Nursebooks.org; 2004.
2. American Nurses Credentialing Center, (ANCC). A subsidiary of the American Nurses Association. Magnet Recognition Program. Recognizing excellence in nursing services application manual. Silver Spring (MD); 2005. p. 14, 80.
3. American Nurses Credentialing Center. Magnet program overview. 2008. Available at: http://www.nursecredentialing.org/Magnet/ProgramOverview.aspx. Accessed July 6, 2008.
4. Aiken LH, Smith HL, Lake ET. Lower Medicare mortality among a set of hospitals known for good nursing care. Med Care 1994;32:771–87.

5. Aiken LH, Sloane DM, Lake ET. Satisfaction with inpatient acquired immunodeficiency syndrome care: a national comparison of dedicated and scattered-bed units. Med Care 1997;36(9):948–62.

6. Kramer M. The magnet hospitals: excellence revisited. J Nurs Adm 1990;20(9):35–44.

7. Kramer M, Schmalenberg C. Job satisfaction and retention insights for the 90's. Nursing 1991;91:50–5.

8. National Database of Nursing Quality Indicators. NDNQI: Transforming data into quality care. 2008. Available at: http://www.nursingquality.org/. Accessed June 25, 2008.

9. National Database of Nursing Quality Indicators. NDNQI: Transforming data into quality care. 2008. Available at: http://www.nursingquality.org/. Accessed July 2, 2008.

10. Registered Nurses' Association of Ontario. Nursing best practice guideline: risk assessment and prevention of pressure ulcers. Toronto: Registered Nurses' Association of Ontario; 2005.

11. Coopey M, Nix MP, Clancy CM. Translating research into evidence-based nursing practice and evaluating effectiveness. J Nurs Care Qual 2006;21(3): 195–200.

12. Pravikoff DS, Tanner AB, Pierce ST. Readiness of U.S. nurses for evidence-based practice: many don't understand or value research and have had little or no training to help them find evidence on which to base their practice. Am J Nurs 2005;105(9):40–52.

13. Sigma Theta Tau International Honor Society of Nursing. 2006 EBP study summary of findings. Available at: http://www.nursingknowledge.org/Portal/CMSLite/Ge. Accessed June 6, 2008.

14. Shamian J. A phenomenal journey, the best practice guidelines project: shaping the future of nursing. RNAO 2007. Toronto: Registered Nurses Association of Ontario.

15. Registered Nurses Association of Ontario. About clinical practice guidelines. Available at: http://www.rnao.org/PageID=1224&SiteNodeID=1588BL_ExpandID=&AA_Shell=. Accessed June 6, 2008.

16. Registered Nurses' Association of Ontario. Spotlight Organizations. 2008. Available at: http://www.rnao.org/Page.asp?PageID=1224&;;SiteNodeID=302. Accessed May 24, 2008.

17. Registered Nurses' Association of Ontario. Toolkit: implementation of clinical practice guidelines. Toronto: Registered Nurses' Association of Ontario; 2002.

18. Ewers K. In-house unpublished evidence-based practice survey. Paper presented at the Clinical Nurse Practice Meeting of Jackson Health System. Miami, Florida, September 22, 2005.

19. Registered Nurses' Association of Ontario. Risk assessment and prevention of pressure ulcers. Toronto: Registered Nurses' Association of Ontario; Revised 2005.

20. Grinspun D, Virani T, Bajnok I. Nursing best practice guidelines: the RNAO project. Healthc Q 2001;5(2): 56–60.

21. Registered Nurses' Association of Ontario. Curricular model for critical care skin champions. Toronto: Registered Nurses' Association of Ontario; 2006.

22. DiCenso A, Virani T, Bajnok I, et al. A toolkit to facilitate the implementation of clinical practice guidelines in health care settings. Hosp Q 2002;5(3): 55–90.

23. Rycroft-Malone J, Harvey G, Kitson A, et al. Getting evidence into practice: ingredients for change. Nurs Stand 2002;16(37):38–43.

24. Davies B, Edwards N, Ploeg J, et al. Determinants of the sustained use of research evidence in nursing: final report. Ottawa (ON): Canadian Health Services Research Foundation and Canadian Institutes fir Health Research; 2006.

25. Registered Nurses' Association of Ontario. Developing and sustaining nursing leadership. Toronto: Registered Nurses' Association of Ontario; 2006. p. 24.

26. Bridges W. Managing transitions. Reading (MA): Addison-Wesley Publishing Company; 1991.

27. Centers for Medicare and Medicaid Services. Incorporating selected National Quality Forum and never events into Medicare's list of hospital-acquired conditions. Available at: http://www.cms.hhs.gov/apps/media/press/factsheet.asp?Counter=3043&;intNumPerPage=1. Accessed July 2, 2008.

28. Registered Nurses' Association of Ontario. Summary of recommendations. Available at: http://www.rnao.org/Storage/12/639/_BPG_Pressure_Ulcers_v2. Accessed May 24, 2008.

29. Edwards N, Davies B, Danseco E, et al. Evaluation of nursing best practice guidelines: perceived worth and educational/supportive processes. CHRU monograph series. Available at: http://rnao.org/researchunit/Storage/22/1641_780_CHRUMonograph_Series_M04-03.pdf. Accessed July 6, 2008.

30. Registered Nurses' Association of Ontario. Assessment and device selection for vascular access. Toronto: Registered Nurses' Association of Ontario; Revised 2008.

31. Registered Nurses' Association of Ontario. Care and maintenance to reduce vascular access complications. Toronto: Registered Nurses' Association of Ontario; Revised 2008.

32. Registered Nurses' Association of Ontario. Prevention of falls and fall injuries in the older adult. Toronto: Registered Nurses' Association of Ontario; Revised 2005.

33. Registered Nurses' Association of Ontario. Women abuse: screening, identification and initial response. Toronto: Registered Nurses' Association of Ontario; 2005.

34. Registered Nurses' Association of Ontario. Embracing cultural diversity in health care: developing cultural competence. Toronto: Registered Nurses' Association of Ontario; 2007.

35. Registered Nurses' Association of Ontario. Collaborative practice among nursing reams guideline. Toronto: Registered Nurses' Association of Ontario; 2006.

36. Registered Nurses' Association of Ontario. Developing and sustaining effective staffing and workload practices. Toronto: Registered Nurses' Association of Ontario; 2007.

37. Ewers K. In-house unpublished evidence-based nursing collaborative curriculum model. Paper presented at the Nursing Forum Seminar at Jackson Health System. Miami, Florida, May 23, 2008.

38. Estabrooks CA, Midodzi WK, Cummings GG, et al. Predicting research use in nursing organizations: a multilevel analysis. Nurse Res 2007;56(4 Suppl):S7–23.

The Virtual ICU (vICU): a New Dimension for Critical Care Nursing Practice

Mary A. Myers, RN, MSN[a],*,
Kevin D. Reed, RN, MSN, NE-BC, CPHQ-BC[b,c]

KEYWORDS

- Virtual intensive care unit • eICU • Technology
- Innovation • Telemedicine • Critical care unit

In its landmark report entitled *Crossing the Quality Chasm: A New Healthcare System for the 21st Century*, the Institute of Medicine reported that health care has safety and quality problems because it relies on outmoded systems of work.[1] The report recommends redesigned systems for health care to achieve higher levels of safety and quality. The virtual or remote ICU (vICU) is a redesigned model of care that uses state-of-the-art technology to leverage the expertise and knowledge of the intensivist and experienced critical care nurse. The model supports the bedside caregiver team in improving patient outcomes over multiple critical care units and large geographic areas. With widespread reports over the past decade that intensivist-led teams and adequate nurse staffing ratios support improved patient outcomes,[2,3] and with the recognition that there is a growing shortage of both, the vICU model of care is gaining increasing national interest.

This article describes the use of vICU technology in the critical care environment and the impact it has on improving quality. It discusses the components of an emerging new practice setting for critical care nurses and describes the many ways that telenursing can impact patient outcomes.

vICU technology or critical care telemedicine in its most advanced form has been compared with air traffic control. In the vICU, specially trained critical care physicians and experienced critical care registered nurses (eRNs) collaborate remotely with the onsite care team to support and enhance the care of critically ill patients. The remote ICU technology tools are designed to support the care process, improving efficiency and effectiveness.[4] The vICU model enables 24/7 care to critical care patients across multiple hospitals using technology to track patients' vital signs and trends. Remote monitoring is supported by software that trends patient information and evaluates bedside monitoring, laboratory, medication, and charted data as they are entered into the bedside clinical information system. The system uses this data to flag situations and issues alerts requiring evaluation by the remote or bedside team.[5] The model is built around preemptive care, in which early interventions support best practices to prevent complications.

Several vendors provide a complete hardware/software/technology product along with services for implementation. The most established company in this market is VISICU.INC, which uses the registered term *eICU* for its system. VISICU was founded in 1998 by Drs. Michael Breslow and Brian Rosenfeld in Baltimore, Maryland.[6] They have placed over 30 systems nationwide

[a] Clarian Inpatient Medicine, Clarian Health, 1800 N Capital, Suite e140, Indianapolis, IN 46202-1252, USA
[b] Adult Critical Care Services, Clarian Health, Methodist Hospital, 1701 N. Senate Boulevard, Room A5237, Indianapolis, IN 46202-1367, USA
[c] American Association of Critical Care Nurses Certification Corporation, Aliso Viejo, CA, USA
* Corresponding author.
E-mail address: mamyers@clarian.org (M. Myers).

Crit Care Nurs Clin N Am 20 (2008) 435–439
doi:10.1016/j.ccell.2008.08.003

since alpha testing was conducted at Sentara Healthcare in Norfolk, Virginia in 2003.[6]

The eICU programs are staffed by board certified intensivists and expert critical care nurses who integrate their education and experience using this technology to provide an extra layer of safety and quality for critically ill patients. Most programs operate with nurses 24 hours a day and physicians 15 to 20 hours per day, 365 days per year, leveraging their expertise as a valuable resource in the current health care climate of increasing patient acuity and decreasing resources. The eICU team has the capability to visually assess patients using high-resolution remote cameras. The cameras have the potential to zoom in close enough to assess a patient's pupils or ventilator settings and to zoom out to visualize nearly the entire patient room. The remote staff converses with bedside staff via a speaker/microphone system installed on the video camera in the patient's room. They also have complete access to the patient's electronic medical record and daily plan of care. By collaborating with the bedside team, the remote ICU team facilitates earlier interventions with the goal of decreasing complications and improving mortality. The bedside team remains the front line of care for the critical care patient while the eICU team is in more of a "supporting role" as a second set of eyes watching out for the safety and quality care of the patient (**Fig. 1**).

CREATING A CULTURE OF COLLABORATION

Use of eICU technology has been associated with improved teamwork and an increased safety climate, especially among nurses.[7] Much of this improvement can be attributed to the eRN's ability to enhance communication among the eICU and bedside ICU staff members to increase

collaborative efforts and build trust. Through the use of eICU technology, the eRN provides real-time communication facilitated by a variety of modalities such as video conferencing, nurse-to-nurse signouts, and hotline telephones to provide instant bi-directional access for bedside clinicians.[6] This communication allows clinical information to flow smoothly through reliable and efficient data management systems. It leads to improved collaboration by connecting sources of information in a seamless process that moves caregivers more quickly toward inquiry and investigation of the causes and interventions for abnormalities that are occurring.

Like anything new, acceptance of the remote ICU will take time, and methodical work must be done to reassure the bedside team that this is not "big brother" checking up on them. It is important that this program is accepted and adopted by the medical and nursing staff in the critical care unit before implementation. Without buy-in and support, it is difficult to achieve the collaboration needed to improve patient care processes.

It is highly recommended that there is a phased plan rollout when implementing this technology across a multi-hospital system. Ensuring that bedside nurses are knowledgeable about how the program can support them is absolutely necessary. Education of the bedside team should include a major focus on the goal of the new model, that is, to back up the front lines and to improve quality and safety of critically ill patients.

Cameras mounted in the patient's room are used for virtual rounding and to assess the patient or situation to see how the eRN or eMD can be of assistance to the bedside staff. These cameras seem to be the most threatening part of the new technology to bedside nurses, and, ironically, they are used the least during the eRN's workflow. Live demonstrations of the vICU in the eICU center can help to alleviate many of the fears associated with the use of the cameras, including spying or taping.

The nurse staffing models used in the eICU include a mix of critical care nurses whose work hours are split between the vICU and a critical care unit and nurses who work exclusively in the vICU. A model in which nurses share their work hours can help tremendously with the acceptance of the program with the bedside team and in marketing the different uses of the eICU. When working at the bedside, the eRN has been able to role model the effective use of the program using their eRN colleague working in the eICU as a consultant and for back-up support. They are also able to remind their peers at the bedside of the availability of intensivist in the eICU at the touch of the eICU button located in every patient room.

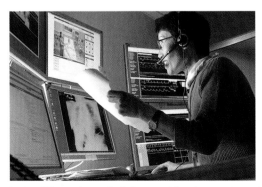

Fig. 1. eRN monitors vital signs and lends an extra set of eyes to patient care. (*Courtesy of* VISICU, Baltimore, MD; with permission.)

With an average of nearly 16 years of critical care experience,[8] eRNs are expert clinicians familiar with evidence-based clinical initiatives that need to occur at the bedside to optimize outcomes for patients. They perform interventions that include issues related to patient safety, follow-up on laboratory values, changes in vital signs, and bedside collaboration with the care team. Many of the eRN interventions are related to patient safety, including proactive measures to prevent errors and complications. Specific interventions include ensuring the correct dosage of intravenous infusions, timely reporting of laboratory values, and compliance with evidenced-based process measures.

Many sites with vICUs allow the medical staff to order a defined level of participation of the virtual or remote ICU team. This aspect can lead to different levels of care and confusion for the nurse in the critical care unit. It is important that the level of ICU telemedicine staff intervention is established and agreed upon before implementation of the technology. It may be necessary to amend medical staff policies and bylaws to reflect that ICU telemedicine is part of the organizational care of critical patients, and that all providers must accept a level of oversight and intervention in the care of their ICU patients.[6]

THE eRN IMPROVING QUALITY AND SAFETY

Incorporation of eICU technology into the care of critically ill patients can greatly improve the structure for quality and safety by enabling improved processes and outcomes. It is not meant to replace the bedside caregiver but to provide a second layer of monitoring and vigilance to strengthen the way work is organized. With a continuous eye on patient vital signs and other clinical data, the eRN is in a unique position to serve as a consultant, collaborating to improve care processes through a consultative role.[8]

Many of the improvements associated with the use of eICU technology can be attributed to improved workflow that ensures adherence to recognized evidenced-based process measures including care bundles. A "bundle" is a collection of process measures needed to effectively and safely care for patients undergoing particular treatments with inherent risks.[9] Several interventions are bundled together and, when used in combination, significantly improve patient care outcomes. Examples include the ventilator bundle, central line bundle, and sepsis bundle. Care bundles are a good starting point for improving care. Because bedside nurses are dealing with multiple complexities and priorities in the environment, the eRN can

be used to track compliance with care bundles to ensure that each process within the bundle is completed. The bundles are considered cohesive units; only when used together do they cause significant improvement.[9]

Care bundle process measures that have been developed include use of the ventilator bundle, which, according to the Institute for Health care Improvement,[9] includes five elements: elevation of the head of the bed (HOB) to 30 to 45 degrees, daily sedation vacation and readiness to extubate, peptic ulcer disease (PUD) prophylaxis, and deep vein thrombosis (DVT) prophylaxis. While completing virtual rounding, the eRN can collaborate with the bedside caregiver to complete a checklist for all patients on a ventilator to ensure compliance with the bundle measures. The patient's HOB is observed for the appropriate elevation, and medical treatment for PUD and DVT is checked against the care plan. This type of process improvement system has been shown to have a statistically significant impact when there is compliance with HOB elevation and DVT and PUD prophylaxis.[10]

In addition to ensuring care bundle compliance, the eRN also monitors other measures associated with improved outcomes. Through the use of protocols and order sets, the eICU team is able to work with the bedside staff to intervene when processes deviate from established standards. For example, the use of a glucose management protocol control has been associated with decreased infection rates and mortality in the critically ill.[11,12] The eRN validates that the appropriate protocols for glucose control are in place and being followed. The eRN accesses blood sugar results and collaborates with the bedside caregiver to adjust insulin dosages. The eRN's expert knowledge of use of the protocol and the interventions needed to ensure that it is strictly adhered to can result in lower average daily glucose levels and improved glucose control.[13]

In addition to evidenced-based care bundles and protocols, the eRN can also be highly effective in screening patients for signs of various complications and can intervene to ensure appropriate treatment is initiated. In one example, evidence suggests that the role of the eRN leads to improved identification of severe sepsis[14] when the outcome of care is highly dependent on early antibiotic therapy.[15] Using specifically designed criteria, patients can be rapidly screened for evidence of severe sepsis, and a care bundle can be initiated immediately. The overall compliance with the implementation of the severe sepsis resuscitation bundle, including each of its elements, may be improved by the use of eICU technology and the eRN's vigilance.[16]

OTHER COMPONENTS OF eRN PRACTICE

The eRN is fully integrated into the care team in the critical care unit and is considered a partner by the bedside staff. As an expert clinician, the eRN fully participates in the development and mentoring of novice critical care nurses by coaching them through difficult patient experiences. Nurses new to the critical care environment can use the eRN to validate assessment findings, critical thinking, and planned interventions. They greatly enhance their ability to have immediate resources available for clinical decision making.[17] In addition, the eRN is available for troubleshooting equipment and providing education about medications, disease processes, standards of care, protocols, and hospital policies and procedures.[18] The ability to access an experienced colleague at any time can be reassuring to a nurse new to the critical care environment. This level of support can help to reduce stress and improve nurse satisfaction and retention.

Use of eICU technology and the eRN can also help to transform performance assessment and improvement initiatives in the critical care environment. Because vICU nurses and physicians provide care over multiple ICUs, they are in a unique position to identify common variances in care. Using virtual technology, they can design reports to produce data about specific patterns they have observed. The detailed information supplied by these sophisticated reports can be used to guide performance improvement activities and monitor their progress.[19] This process enhances the ability for performance improvement initiatives to be implemented, monitored, and standardized for best practices across multiple units to promote quality and safety.[19] The eRN is in an optimal position to assist in developing, implementing, and expanding best practice standards to achieve uniformity.[20]

FUTURE IMPLICATIONS

The University Health Consortium recently evaluated ICU remote technology and reported that ICU telemedicine will likely be a standard of care in critical care units in 10 years. This finding suggests that all hospitals should begin now to evaluate budget, staffing, technology, and infrastructure needs for future eICU implementation.[21] In addition to its use in critical units, the technology includes portable vICU work stations that can be used to connect critically ill patients in emergency rooms, labor and delivery, and medical-surgical units to the vICU bunker to gain oversight access by an intensivist and eRN. Currently, several hospitals are taking this technology beyond the walls of the critical care unit. It is rapidly being implemented in progressive and intermediate care units where nurse-to-patient ratios are higher and patients continue to need close observation and surveillance. Some vICUs have leveraged pharmacist (PharmD) support from the center to provide rural hospitals with night pharmacy resources, an otherwise unaffordable option.

A virtual care delivery system opens endless possibilities for the future. In the medical-surgical unit, this technology could be used as leveraging a "concierge service" whereby a service worker makes regularly scheduled rounds to ask the patient whether there is anything they can get for them. It can also be connected to the patient call button so there is an immediate response via two-way video with a service worker's smiling face asking, "How can I assist you?" The e-hospital version of the remote ICU includes nurses and hospitalists conducting virtual rounds on medical-surgical patients to ensure safe quality care.

SUMMARY

The eICU has redefined the care delivery model, supporting higher quality and safer care. It is imperative that all health care leaders continue to think "out of the box" on how to use this technology in their critical care units and beyond. Much like air traffic controllers monitoring airplanes with passengers, this technology facilitates remote nurses and physicians to monitor a hospital's sickest patient, ensuring safe passage to their destination.

REFERENCES

1. Institute of Medicine Committee on the Quality of Healthcare in America, Richardson WC, Berwick DM, et al. Crossing the quality chasm: a new healthcare system for the 21st century. Washington (DC): National Academy Press; 2001.
2. Jean-Louis V. Need for intensivists in intensive care units. Lancet 2000;356:695–6.
3. Tranow-Mordi WO, Hau C, Warden A, et al. Hospital mortality in relation to staff workload: a 4 year study in an adult intensive care unit. Lancet 2000;356: 185–9.
4. Celi LA, Hassan E, Marquardt C, et al. The eICU: it's not just telemedicine. Crit Care Med 2001;29(8): 183–9.
5. Breslow MJ. Remote ICU care programs: current status. J Crit Care 2007;22:67–8.

6. VISICU. Technology improved care for the 21st century. Available at: http://www.visicu.com. Accessed May 31, 2008.

7. Thomas EJ, Chu-Weininger MYL, Lucke J, et al. The impact of a tele-ICU on provider attitudes about teamwork and safety culture. Crit Care Med 2007; 35(12):A25.

8. American Association of Critical Care Nurses Certification Corporation. A national practice analysis of nurses working in the virtual intensive care unit, 2006.

9. Institute for Healthcare Improvement. Bundle up for safety. Available at: http://www.ihi.org/IHI/Topics/CriticalCare/IntensiveCare/ImprovementStories. Accessed June 2, 2008.

10. Youn BA. ICU process improvement: using telemedicine to enhance compliance and documentation for the ventilator bundle. Chest 2006; 130:226C.

11. Krinsley JS. Effect of an intensive glucose management protocol on the mortality of critically ill adult patients. Mayo Clin Proc 2005;80(8):1101.

12. Institute for Healthcare Improvement. Improving glucose control: ICU and beyond. Available at: http://www.ihi.org/IHI/Topics/CriticalCare/Improvement Stories. Accessed June 2, 2008.

13. Aaronson ML, Zawada ET Jr, Herr P. Role of telemedicine intensive care unit program on glycemic control in seriously ill patients in a rural health system. Chest 2006;130:226A.

14. Rincon T, Ikeda D, Seiver A. Screening for severe sepsis: an incidence analysis. Crit Care Med 2007; 35(12):A257.

15. Institute for Healthcare Improvement. Implement the sepsis resuscitation bundle: improve time to broad spectrum antibiotics. Available at: http://www.hih.org/IHI/Topics/CriticalCare/Sepsis/Changes/Individual Changes/ImproveTim. Accessed June 1, 2008.

16. Patel B, Kao L, Thomas E, et al. Improving compliance with surviving sepsis campaign guidelines via remote electronic ICU monitoring. Crit Care Med 2007;35(12):A275.

17. Rufo RJZ. Virtual ICU's: foundations for healthier work environments. Nurs Manage 2007;38(2):32–9.

18. Witzke AK. Trends in telemedicine. Men in Nursing 2007;2(1):46–54.

19. VISICU. Core reports. Available at: http://www.visicu.com/products/evantagesoftware/reports. Accessed June 3, 2008.

20. McCauley K, Irwin RS. Changing the work environment in intensive care units to achieve patient-focused care: the time has come. Am J Crit Care 2006;15(6):541–7.

21. Cummings JP. UHC technology report: intensive care telemedicine March 2006. Available at: http://uhc.edu/publications. Accessed June 1, 2008.

Working in an eICU Unit: Life in the Box

Trudi B. Stafford, RN, PhD[a,b,*], Mary A. Myers, RN, MSN[c],
Anne Young, RN, EdD[a], Janet G. Foster, RN, PhD[a],
Jeffrey T. Huber, PhD[d]

KEYWORDS

- eICU • eNurse • ePhysician • eClinician
- VISICU • Telemedicine

The VISICU eICU model of care (VISICU, Inc., Baltimore, MD) offers a telemedicine platform that allows intensivists and experienced intensive care unit (ICU) nurses to monitor many ICU patients continuously from a remote location. Note that eICU is a trade symbol and is not an abbreviation for a set of words. The eICU model of care is a new approach to maximizing the advantage of intensivist medical management of ICU patients at a time when a nation-wide shortage of intensivists exists. Approximately 40 eICU programs exist across the nation.[1] The work environment of the eICU team (eTeam) is physically removed from the ICU setting, with health care workers in the eICU unit having no "hands-on" experiences with the patients they monitor. This remote work environment is unique to medical disciplines that have historically been "hands on." The purpose of this article is to share the findings of an ethnographic study that describes what it is like to work in the eICU environment.

Telemedicine is defined as the delivery of health care services across a distance, with health care professionals "using information and communications technologies for the exchange of valid information for diagnosis, treatment and prevention of disease and injuries, research and evaluation, and for the continuing education of health care providers, all in the interest of advancing the health of individuals and their communities."[2] The eICU model of care is a form of telemedicine that was developed in an effort to use state-of-the-art technology to provide intensivist-driven care even when it is not possible to have an intensivist at the bedside.[3,4]

Previous studies of the eICU model of care mainly focused on quantitative elements, evaluating specific clinical outcomes rather than examining the way such units function. Issues such as cost effectiveness and reduction of morbidity and mortality brought about these studies to justify the creation of these units. Rosenfeld and colleagues[3] evaluated the feasibility of using telemedicine to provide 24-hour intensivist oversight as a means of improving clinical outcomes for ICU patients. This triple-cohort, observational, time-series study occurred in a 10-bed surgical ICU in an academic-affiliated community hospital. Evaluations of mortality, severity-adjusted hospital complications, and economic factors were made by comparing two 16-week study periods before eICU model of care implementation with a 16-week period following intervention. Findings revealed that severity-adjusted ICU mortality and severity-adjusted hospital complications decreased significantly during the intervention

[a] Texas Woman's University, College of Nursing, 6700 Fannin Street, Houston, TX 77030, USA
[b] Patient Care Services, University of Pittsburgh Medical Center – Passavant/Passavant Cranberry, 9100 Babcock Boulevard, Pittsburgh, PA 15237, USA
[c] Clarian Inpatient Medicine Program, Clarian Health Systems, 1800 N. Capital, Suite e140, Indianapolis, IN 46202-1252, USA
[d] Texas Woman's University, School of Library and Information Studies, 6700 Fannin Street, Houston, TX 77030, USA
* Corresponding author. University of Pittsburgh Medical Center – Passavant/Passavant Cranberry, 9100 Babcock Boulevard, Pittsburgh, PA 15237.
E-mail address: staffordtb@upmc.edu (T.B. Stafford).

Crit Care Nurs Clin N Am 20 (2008) 441–450
doi:10.1016/j.ccell.2008.08.013

period. The incidence of ICU complications also decreased significantly. Although the ICU length of stay decreased, hospital length of stay showed no significant difference. Costs associated with the reduced ICU length of stay decreased by one third. The investigators concluded that the eICU model of care was a viable program for remote monitoring of ICU patients, offering improved quality of care and decreasing ICU costs for units that did not have on-site 24-hour intensivist coverage.

To evaluate whether eICU programs could improve clinical and economic outcomes across multiple ICUs, Breslow and colleagues[5] conducted a before-and-after trial using two adult ICUs in a 650-bed tertiary care teaching hospital. The study included a total of 2140 patients who received ICU care between 1999 and 2001 before implementation (n = 1396) and after implementation (n = 744). The eTeam provided supplemental remote monitoring and management of patients for 19 hours per day (12:00 noon to 7:00 AM). Findings indicated that hospital mortality for ICU patients was lower during the implementation period. ICU length of stay was shorter during the time period when the eICU model of care was in place. Economically, variable costs per case were lower and hospital revenues were higher, primarily from increased case volumes. Shorter length of stay decreased cost per case and created the capacity to increase the number of ICU cases per month by increasing the monthly contribution margin.

The findings from these studies encouraged further development of eICU programs. The eICU model of care represents a new mechanism for effective care delivery. It requires an interface between onsite and remote care providers. To date, no published studies describe the eICU work environment from the perspective of health care workers employed in that setting. The purpose of this ethnographic study was to describe the experiences of the health care workers in the eICU department and to examine how health care workers function in this setting.

PHILOSOPHIC UNDERPINNINGS

The philosophic orientation of symbolic interactionism guided this study. Symbolic interactionism focuses on social interactions to explain human behavior and thought.[6] Symbolic interactionism involves a process of "communication, role taking, self direction, and ongoing adjustment that is an essential part of what people are."[7] It shapes the identities of people and the society in which they live. To understand the society of the eICU work environment, one must understand the symbolic interactions that take place among the members

of the eTeam in their work environment. Interactions observed in the eICU unit were analyzed according the following categories: role taking, communicating, interpreting one another, adjusting one's acts to one another, directing and controlling self, and sharing perspectives.

METHODS

Ethnography provides a detailed, in-depth description of everyday life and practice.[8] It is a research methodology whereby the ethnographer (researcher) interacts directly with the people who are being studied to allow them to tell their own stories.[9] The product of the research is a constructed reality that is derived from varying viewpoints of the observer and those observed.[10] The ethnographer is the interpreter of "multiple voices and experiences,"[11] using the words of those being studied and the observations made during the field study to capture and describe the essence of the experience being studied.

Human subject approval was obtained from the participating institutions' institutional review boards. Following informed consent, the principal investigator interacted with the eTeam during field study in the unit on weekdays, evenings, and weekends by sitting alongside health care workers in the unit. Interactions between the principal investigator and the eTeam during the field study and interviews caused no disruption in patient care. Semistructured interviews regarding activities, observations, or validation of findings were conducted, with individual members of the eTeam in concurrence with the field observations.

Fieldwork involved 60 hours of observation of activities associated with work in the eICU department. Observations were used to learn about how the unit functioned, to confirm those activities that were described during the personal interviews, and to identify activities needing further investigation. Observations in the eICU department occurred in multiple blocks of time to encompass different times of day and night to capture various staffing matrices. The eICU department is staffed with eICU nurses (eNurses) around the clock, 7 days a week. Intensivists are not included in the staffing matrix for the entire 24 hours of every day. The researcher conducted fieldwork during time periods with staffing matrices that included and did not include intensivists. Team dynamics were observed according to these varying staffing matrices.

Field notes were transcribed within 1 week of completion of the fieldwork, with interviews recorded and transcribed to written text within 1 week of the interview. Any names or identifiers used during interviews were eliminated during the transcription. Identified themes were tracked by way of an audit trail and confirmed with the eICU personnel throughout the data collection period.

Trustworthiness was established by ensuring credibility, transferability, dependability, and confirmability. Credibility was established through a comprehensive description that accurately described the information gathered in personal interviews with the eICU staff and extensive time spent observing the staff working in the eICU department. Transferability was ensured through triangulation of the sources of the data.[12] In this study, concurrent analysis of findings occurred when interviews and fieldwork were ongoing to ensure dependability. Some participants were interviewed and observed more than once to validate findings. Emerging categories and supporting data were verified with eICU staff to confirm the validity of the emerging themes. This process, along with audit trails, ensured confirmability.[12]

Setting

The setting for this study was an eICU department known as the eCollaborative, located in Metropolitan Hospital, the flagship institution in the Good Shepherd Health Care System (GSHC) (all names used are pseudonyms), a large health care system in the midwestern United States. Established less than 3 years before this study, this unit was responsible for monitoring 180 ICU beds located in four hospitals around a large metropolitan area. All patients admitted to these ICU beds were automatically monitored by the eTeam.

Sample

This study included a purposive sample of all eNurses and eICU physicians (ePhysicians) working in the eICU department. All eICU staff members have worked at the bedside in ICUs before working in the eICU unit and all were invited to participate in this study. Currently, 44 eICU registered nurses (eRNs), 26 ePhysicians, and two information technology staff members make up the eTeam. Thirteen eNurses, three ePhysicians, and one information technology systems analyst participated in semistructured interviews, and 27 additional eICU clinicians (eClinicians) participated in the field study. All eClinicians have worked at the bedside in ICUs before working in the eICU unit. Years of clinical experience and experience in critical care for this sample ranged from 5 years to more than 30 years. Some of the eNurses continue to work at least one shift per week at the bedside in an ICU. Educational preparation for the eNurses ranged from associate's degree to master's degree with several eNurses currently pursuing advanced degrees.

Analysis of Data

Data collection and analysis proceeded concurrently. Transcribed interviews and participant observations were analyzed for descriptive comments about the eICU work environment and the relationships among those working in the eICU department. Statements found in the interview transcripts were clustered into categories. Emerging categories were clarified by observation in the field study and verbal confirmation from the participants. A process of coding, memos, and typologizing ensured the capture of pertinent categories.[13]

WORKING IN THE "BOX"

The eNurses and intensivists (ePhysicians) conduct their work in a centralized location, which is affectionately known as the "CORE," the "Bunker," or the "Box." The physical appearance of the eICU department can be intimidating initially because of the massive amount of technology in a limited space. The Box, a single room (700 square feet) housed within one of the hospitals, contains eight computer stations. The unit is staffed with six eNurses and one ePhysician, who work from these computer stations. Each computer station has a desk that easily moves up and down to allow one to work both sitting and standing. Each work station has a multiple-line telephone, along with two computers, two keyboards, two pointing devices or mice, one headset with an earpiece and microphone, and a total of six to eight screens. Although the appearance may be intimidating, eClinicians break it down to make it seem more manageable. One of the eNurses explained, "I think sometimes some people are really intimidated because it looks like, oh, my gosh, you've got six computer screens and you narrow it down to say well it's really only two computers."

Experiences differ in the Box during the day and night shifts. By day, the Box is well lit and the front door to the unit is propped open. It is not unusual for unannounced tours, hospital leaders, students, equipment and drug representatives, and nurses orienting to the ICU to drop into the unit. In contrast, by night, lights in the department are turned down. At change of shift, one of the eNurses announced as she turned down the lights, "Now, it is officially the night shift." Rarely does anyone other than members of the eTeam visit the unit on the night shift. Monica, an eNurse who works both day and night shifts, stated, "On the day shift, it is open house. On the night shift, it is by invitation only." As a result, conversations and activities are more reserved during the day shift than on the night shift.

A Different World: eICU Relationships and Encounters

Relationships and encounters that occur within the eTeam and between the eTeam and the bedside team are often worlds apart. The working relationship among the members of the eTeam can be described as esprit de corps. The individual eNurses and ePhysicians function as a true team.

Open communication was observed during the field study. The close proximity of those working in the Box has a big impact on the climate and collegiality of the work environment. The eTeam often uses humor and statements made for shock value as the members interact with one another. As the day shift winds down and the risk for having someone from administration or the outside pop in the unit for an unannounced visit is decreased, the banter among the eTeam is more spirited. Conversation topics run the gamut from personal to professional and most eTeam members join in the conversations. No walls exist between the computer stations. The eTeam works in close quarters, with little privacy. Most conversations within the unit and on the telephone are overheard by all in the Box. During both the day shift and the night shift, one can hear the members of the eTeam conversing with each other socially and professionally. eNurse-to-eTeam consultations regarding patient issues are common.

The eTeam members admit that they all have "strong personalities." Donna, an eNurse, describes the strong personalities of the eNurses collectively as "a stable of alpha dogs."

Donna further elaborates, "The problem is that you can't get away from issues that you find irritating. You can't go run and hide in your patient's room because you don't have a patient room to run into." As a result, the eTeam members resolve personality conflicts and issues among themselves in real time to avoid tension in the workplace. Steven, an eNurse, commented, "If we have a problem with a coworker, we say it and resolve it right away."

The eNurses and ePhysicians are complimentary of each other and the value that their roles bring to the entire eTeam. Both disciplines believe they have unique and positive relationships that are different from those relationships at the bedside. Madison, an eNurse, shared, "I do think that we have a unique relationship with our physicians who work here. They're really a big part of our team. We are not afraid to bring anything to

their attention and ask them anything or to explain something to us or whatever. It's kind of like they're just one of us when they're sitting there. They are just very much just one of the gang." One of the ePhysicians reciprocated, "The eNurses are great, with lots of experience."

ePhysicians and eNurses verbally expressed their respect for one another based on their interactions with each other and the respect for the knowledge and experience that each individual brings to the team. All eTeam members have a minimum of 5 years of bedside ICU experience in an ICU specialty such as cardiovascular, neurology, or surgical care. Most eTeam members were modest about the talent they bring to the team but instead talked about the fact that they depend heavily on each other to answer any questions that might be raised by the bedside team. They were observed acting as instant resources of information to other eTeam members. Donna, one of the eNurses with a lengthy history of neurology ICU experience, recognized that the bedside team may call her with questions outside its area of expertise and outside or within her area of expertise. Again, realizing that she may not know the answer to the bedside nurse's question, Donna went on to say, "Typically, there is someone sitting in this room [the Box] with the expertise to help you answer the question."

Physical and Mental Stressors: an Unexpected Discovery

As eNurses transitioned into the telemedicine work environment, they found physical stressors related to this work environment that were unforeseen.

One of the eNurses rubbed her neck as she complained that she gets a recurring pain in her upper back from repeatedly using the computer mouse. Another eNurse commented that her neck hurts from the angle of the monitors. She has learned over time to keep her work table low and her chair high to avoid discomfort. Two eNurses have had carpal tunnel syndrome surgery but further investigation shows that the repetitive injury associated with this syndrome occurred before these nurses began working in the eICU department. Several eNurses admitted to having had bloodshot eyes daily when they first started working as eNurses. At least one had glasses prescribed with antireflection and magnification. After a while, she forgot to wear them and now she never wears them. One eNurse wears gloves while she works because she has developed a contact dermatitis since working in the eICU department.

Although physical stress was a main reason for some to leave the bedside work environment, the eICU work environment is the extreme opposite. The lack of physical activity in this new work environment has its own challenges. Weight gain, fatigue, boredom, and lack of ability to concentrate are common side effects of the lack of movement by the eTeam. One eNurse describes the weight gain when someone joins the eTeam as the "freshman 15." In an effort to combat the weight gain due to the change in activity levels in this new work environment, the eNurses initiated a weight-loss program affectionately known as "the biggest loser" that has shown a great deal of success in weight control for the eTeam.

Frequently, on any given shift, whether it be day or night shift, it is not uncommon to hear a member of the eTeam say, "I'm sleepy." The eTeam members help each other combat the fatigue. Someone may suggest that the sleepy person stand up to do his/her work or may offer him/her a cup of coffee.

Boredom comes from the repetitive work-related activities that are inherent in the role of continuously monitoring patients by rounding on each of them according to his/her level of acuity. The lack of ability to concentrate happens when one works on the computer for long periods of time without breaks. As one eNurse described it, "Your brain gets fuzzy if you look at the computer screen for too long." Distractions and frequent breaks are encouraged to fight the boredom and lack of ability to concentrate. Given that each eTeam member has a pod partner, it is easy to take breaks without compromising patient care. All of the eNurses and ePhysicians bring in items to facilitate distraction. One eNurse referred to the various personal backpacks and bags around the Box as their "bag of tricks." These bags contain things like magazines, bills that need to be paid, books, food items, and other personal items. Diversion plays an important role in maintaining mental sharpness while at the computer.

For some, food fulfills a diversionary role in the eCollaborative work experience. Food is frequently out on the table and all who enter the Box are welcome to partake in whatever happens to be available. eNurses freely admit, "Most of the food that is brought to the hospital by drug reps ends up here." Another eNurse chimes in, "You can get lots to eat if you stay around here for any length of time."

Some eTeam members keep one of their computer screens on a non–work-related Web site to have a distraction at eye's view at all times. Others periodically walk away from the computer station to "clear their heads." They visit with one another in the unit or they walk outside of the unit for a fresh perspective. When an eNurse leaves the Box, his/her eNurse pod partner pulls up a screen to monitor the alarms on his/her patients to watch them while he/she is off of the unit. Occasionally, visitors to the unit provide a much-needed distraction. One evening, a chaplain brought in one of her service dogs for a visit. She stated, "This is a stress reliever for the staff."

Walking on Eggshells: eTeam/Bedside Team Interaction

The experiences of interacting with the bedside team while working in the eICU work environment were more strained. The goal of communication between the eTeam and the bedside team is to share information in an effort to provide the highest quality of patient care. Effective interaction between the eTeam and bedside team is critical to the success of the eICU model of care because the eTeam can only make recommendations of actions to be taken by the bedside team, given that the eTeam is operating from a remote location away from the patients. The eTeam described the interaction process with the bedside team as "walking on eggshells." As Anne, the eICU nursing director, explained, "Communication [is] the number one skill" that is necessary in encounters between the bedside ICU team and the eTeam. The eTeam takes ownership of ensuring that all communications are professional, nonjudgmental, and nonoffensive toward its bedside counterparts.

Melissa, the eICU clinical manager, identified collaborative communication for the good of the patient as paramount in training bedside clinicians to work in the eICU work environment. She recognized that teaching effective communication skills is ongoing. She stated, "The communication skills are something you just have to work with continuously." She further explained, "We didn't know what we didn't know at the time! You learn over time what things offend people. We spent lots of time in training on communication skills and in discussions about how to phrase things." She gave a specific example: "Saying, 'Did you know the potassium is high?' comes across much differently than, 'I was checking in; I got a result back; may I share it with you?' The same message comes across two very different ways." The eTeam spent a great deal of time talking about collaborative communication skills needed when all communication with the bedside team would not be face to face. Melissa went on to say, "I think the other thing that assists the eNurses with effective communication is that two thirds of them still work at the bedside. I think that's important for both bedside team and the eTeam. It's important for the bedside team to know that the eTeam members really know what it's like out there in the trenches."

Melissa and Anne both emphasized that polishing communication skills never stops for the eTeam because "there is always a way that you can communicate better and always somebody who's going to be offended by the way you said something."

Some interactions between the eTeam and the bedside team occur over the camera in the patient's room. Standards were developed by the eTeam and the bedside team to limit the amount of time that the eICU cameras are on in the patient's room to decrease the perception by the bedside team members that they are being watched. The discomfort of feeling as if they were being watched by the eTeam is a common complaint expressed by the bedside team members. As a result, camera time is monitored by eCollaborative leadership. Camera etiquette standards have been developed to include ringing a bell in the room when the camera is activated, and the eTeam member introducing him/herself and stating the purpose of activating the camera, and then announcing when he/she is turning off the camera. Those eNurses and ePhysicians who do not follow the camera standards are counseled and are subject to disciplinary actions for repetitive noncompliance with the standards.

As far as communicating, Madison, an eNurse, shared, "You just have to get a feel for how to communicate with the bedside team. The camera is what scares people most of all, including talking over the camera." Steven, an eNurse on the night shift, shared how he communicates with the bedside team: "Well, with the bedside nurses, I just try to be very gentle with my suggestions. I make suggestions versus orders because I'm not their boss. I tell them something I'm seeing and what I would or would not do that might keep the patients safer or help them get better quicker."

Some of the bedside team members respond well to communications by the eTeam; however, others do not reciprocate with the same collaborative communication style back to the eTeam. Madison explains, "It's not always the long-term nurses, but usually the ones with a chip on their shoulder, who are rude in how they speak to us. Those nurses feel like they know what they're doing and they don't need somebody watching them. What they don't realize is that we're not really watching them, we're watching the patient." She further elaborates, "We're tracking and trending what's going on to make sure our patients are safe. If people could just come to grips with that, then everybody would just be okay." Madison goes on to say, "It [communications with the bedside team] has gotten much, much better over time. But in the beginning it was really, really rough." Melissa, an eNurse, admitted, "Probably the biggest error we continue to make is ticking people off."

Some resentment has occurred in the past on the part of the ICU team that may account for some of the less-than-collaborative communications from the bedside team directed toward the eClinicians. When nurses were recruited to work on the eTeam, it left some units short staffed. One of the ePhysicians recalled that some felt that the ICUs were being "raided" of the most experienced and best ICU nurses to staff the eICU department. Some of the bedside nurses looked on the eNurses as defectors from bedside practice and questioned their commitment to the field of nursing. Donna, an eNurse who also continues to work shifts at the bedside, recalls a conversation she had after working a shift in the ICU with a bedside nurse, Monica. In the parking garage, Monica said to Donna, "Oh, you worked as a real nurse tonight." Donna went on to say, "I told her that I am a real nurse every night." Preserving the credibility of the eNurses and the ePhysicians is paramount. eNurses are encouraged to work shifts at the bedside in ICUs that are monitored by the eCollaborative. It is believed that the members of the bedside team will have more respect and improved communication with the eNurses when they work side-by-side with them at the bedside.

The learning curve for collaborative communication between the eTeam and the bedside team has been steep. Ongoing communication skills are carefully monitored and practiced continuously. All eTeam members and hospital leadership attest that vast improvements in effective communication for the benefit of good patient care have been recognized over time. Anne states, "Many of the eNurses are very skilled with assertive, nonthreatening communication that makes a positive difference in patient care. Our seasoned eNurses do this well."

No Substitution for Bedside Caregivers: Supporting the Onsite Team

The eTeam functions in a supporting, versus starring, role in the patient care experience. The value and return on investment the eTeam brings are improved patient outcomes through improving patient safety and improving quality of care, and cost avoidance by preventing errors and reducing complications associated with ICU stays. The eTeam functions in a passive or active intervention mode. In the passive mode, the eClinician awaits contact from the bedside team to offer assistance. In the active mode, the eClinician has identified an intervention that requires a specific patient interaction on the part of the bedside clinician.

The eNurse functions primarily as an "in-house counsel," one who is available to the bedside team for consultation, exchange of information, and suggestions for actions to be taken by the bedside ICU team. The eNurse is a resource to the ICU nurses and physicians who answers specific patient-related questions, researches patient information from the electronic medical record, and looks up general information (Google is a favorite search engine). Historically, eNurses were specialized ICU nurses before joining the eTeam. In the eICU work environment, they have had to move to a generalist role rather than a specialist role because they monitor many different ICUs that cover many different medical specialties.

Donna discussed how eNurses function in the context of the global patient care team. She indicated her function is not unlike a "virtual charge nurse who knows pertinent information about many patients instead of every minute detail about the care of two ICU patients." Most of her interactions with the bedside team involve discussions about specific patient issues. She explained that most of the questions she gets from the bedside team are those that would normally go to the charge nurse on the unit. As Donna put it, "The computers and the cameras are great tools, but the most important thing we do is provide the bedside team with instant access to an experienced ICU nurse [eNurse] or an intensivist [ePhysician] when they need it." Donna expressed that one of her greatest satisfactions as an eNurse is when she can support a new ICU nurse who would normally have to rely on access to the ICU charge nurse for guidance.

The skill set used by the eNurses is not unlike the skills used at the bedside. One of the eNurses, Madison, said, "You're still using all the same information you used at the bedside; you're just using it in a different way. You're using that same basic assessment of a patient and your critical care nurse thinking skills to know appropriate and best care for the patients. You look at the patient's orders, results of their [diagnostic] tests, and how they are doing."

The eNurse rounds on patients remotely, according to the patient's acuity. The acuity system is color coded as red for the highest acuity, yellow for moderate acuity, and green or an eyeball icon as the lowest acuity. The frequency of rounding is dictated by the acuity scale. Patients who have an acuity rating of red are rounded on every hour. Patients of lesser acuity, with a yellow rating, are rounded on every 2 hours, and patients who are rated green or eyeball are rounded on every 4 hours.

In addition to rounding, the eNurse responds to alerts that pop on the computer screen that indicate a change in a patient's condition. Changes in the patient's condition pop up by way of the VIS-ICU decision support system in the form of Smart Alerts.[14] These alerts are identified by patient and a color-coded severity system, with red as the most severe and requiring immediate attention, yellow as moderately severe, and green as a minor severity. When an alert pops up on the eNurse's screen, the eNurse uses the mouse to pull up the patient's historical and current hemodynamic status and to determine if the alarm is real or artifact. The role of the eNurse is to troubleshoot for possible reasons for the alarm. Once the reason for the alarm is identified, the alarm is dismissed and reset by the eNurse. If the eNurse is unable to clarify the reason for the alarm, the eNurse will camera into the patient's ICU room to visualize the patient and identify if the bedside nurse is working with the patient and is aware of the alarm. The eNurse will consult with the bedside nurse as needed to either dismiss the alarm or determine if a bedside intervention is necessary. If no member of the bedside team is in the room when the eNurse activates the camera and the alarm is real, the eNurse will notify the bedside nurse of the situation by telephone. If the eNurse cannot reach the bedside nurse in a timely manner, the eNurse will contact the bedside charge nurse.

When the ePhysician is in the Box, he/she is viewed by the eNurses and bedside nurses as "Johnny-on-the-spot." The ePhysician is instantly available as an information resource and another set of eyes to assess the patient visually. The ePhysician has the ability to write orders, run codes until the bedside team is in place, and read and interpret diagnostic tests. The eNurses report "an increase in the number of phone calls we receive from the bedside nurses when the doctor comes on duty." Some even perceive that the bedside nurses, at times, hold on to issues until the ePhysician is on duty rather than hunt down the resident or attending physician for orders. The ePhysicians do not all share that perception. The ePhysician generally only rounds on those patients known by the ePhysician or those who have been identified as high acuity who are exhibiting deteriorating trends in vital signs. The role of the ePhysician in regards to patient alerts is to offer advice and consultation, including issuing orders to the bedside team in the absence of the attending physician.

ePhysicians do experience a sense of limitation when off site. Dr. Morgan, one of the ePhysicians, explained the main limitations of providing intensivist coverage from afar: "There are basically two reasons why an ICU needs intensivist coverage: to insert central lines and to intubate patients. Neither of these can be done by the eICU physician. We still have to have someone available in the unit to perform these actions."

During one code, the ePhysician was observed communicating with the bedside team and ran the code until physicians arrived at the bedside. Then, the ePhysician communicated a brief history of the event to the bedside physician, offered assistance, and then quietly monitored the situation through the camera for the duration of the code. The ePhysician explained why he remains quiet once the bedside team is in place: "They know I am here if they need me."

Nurses also experience the frustration that can build when unable to intervene in a hands-on capacity. Even when intervening in an active mode, eNurses must wait for the bedside nurse to complete the requested assessment or carry out the suggestion. Sense of time passage is a significant factor. Steven, an eNurse, explained some of his frustrations while patiently waiting on the bedside nurse to take action on a suggested intervention to address a patient's changing condition: "Time moves more slowly when you are watching through the camera. You have to remember that time is moving much faster for the bedside nurse. She has more than one patient, families, and others to deal with, and many more things that are pulling her away from the patient." He explains, "I have to be understanding of that on my end. If the patient is in danger and the nurse has not intervened, then I will escalate up to the charge nurse. But, if the patient is in no immediate danger, I wait for the nurse to address the situation."

Even recognizing the time factor, a sense of urgency still exists to ensure that suggested actions are taken. Donna, a seasoned ICU nurse turned eNurse, says, "Sometimes I just want to jump through that camera and take action myself. It can be hard to wait on the nurse to take action." Madison, another eNurse, states, "Some days I feel more stressed than others, depending on what unit I'm watching. There may be a charge nurse who does not really understand what you're saying but you feel like there is something that really needs to be done [for the patient]. That can be stressful because you don't have robot arms to reach through the camera and take care of the issue yourself."

The bedside team definitely drives the patient care experience. The eTeam has no hands-on contact with patients and is connected with the bedside team by way of computers, cameras, and telephones. The nature of the eICU work environment can cause frustration. All of the eTeam members were once accomplished bedside clinicians. One ePhysician described his frustration in watching a code from the view of the camera: "You can do everything you could do in the room with your hands tied behind your back." Hence, clear communication and collaboration with the bedside team are needed because they are "your hands" on the patient.

One evening during rounds, the eNurse noticed that a patient was acting restless and trying to get out of bed. No alarms were triggered, even though her nasal oxygen cannula was not in place. To the eNurse, it appeared that the patient might be exhibiting behaviors not uncommon with respiratory distress and oxygen starvation. The eNurse asked the ePhysician on duty to visualize the patient from his computer station. After assessing the patient through the camera, the ePhysician agreed that the behavior was consistent with lack of adequate oxygenation. The ePhysician and the eNurse communicated with the patient by way of the camera to ask if she was okay and to ask her to put her nasal oxygen cannula back in place. She did not respond verbally and did not reposition her oxygen tubing. The ePhysician called the bedside nurse and asked that she go to the patient's room to do an assessment. The ePhysician and eNurse monitored the situation through the camera until the bedside nurse indicated that the patient was not in respiratory distress. The nurse explained that the patient had a history of exhibiting similar behavior in an effort to get attention because she had no visitors and was lonely. As the ePhysician restated the obvious, "There is only so much we can do through a camera. There is no substitution for the bedside caregiver."

Cost Avoidance in the eICU Model of Care

Initially, eICU units had to justify their existence. Based on prior studies, cost effectiveness, reduced length of stay, and decreased mortality were criteria used to justify the cost of an eICU programs. These measures, however, were unable to demonstrate the effectiveness anticipated, so alternate factors that more specifically addressed the function of the eICU program were examined. The eICU nursing director developed the interventions log, which lists passive and active interventions, as a means of reporting on the benefits of the eICU model of care to facility and hospital system executives. As the eICU program began, Anne collected data in the hopes of showing decreased length of stay and decreased mortality rates for ICU patients monitored by the eTeam. Anne noted, "I realized that I was not going to be able to show that we were decreasing length of stay. I started asking my colleagues across the country if they had decreased length of stay and many confirmed that they had not decreased length of stay." She recalls, "I didn't know how much pressure I was going to be under to keep my program running, so I quickly evaluated that the true value in this service was all of the interventions that are happening by these fabulous nurses in the eICU unit. So we started logging them. In looking at the log, we were able to show that we were preventing patient harm. We had identified errors that had occurred and we had prevented potential errors from happening. We realized that we had to use these interventions to communicate what GSHS was getting for their investment." As one of the ePhysicians confirmed, "The eCollaborative is not a money maker. Its value is in cost avoidance."

Anne specifically used the interventions log in speaking with the chief nursing officer from one of the community hospitals. Six ICU beds had been monitored by the eTeam for about a year. Anne explained, "I knew I would never have enough data in 10 years to show that we decreased their length of stay or we'd even decreased their mortality. I went to her and said I can't show you that we've decreased mortality and I can't show you we've decreased length of stay, but I can share with you the interventions attributed to the eNurses and ePhysicians. I believe that if we turn this [eICU model of care] off tomorrow we would be affecting the quality and safety of your patients." Anne read examples of actual interventions that were initiated by the eTeam on patients in this hospital's ICU. By the time Anne read the third example of an intervention, the chief nursing officer "was sold" on the value of the eICU model of care and is now a staunch supporter. From then on, Anne, Dr. Young, and Melissa have continued to use the interventions log to justify the value of the eICU model of care.

SUMMARY

According to Madison, one of the eNurses, working in the eICU department is like working in air traffic control. One works in front of a computer screen monitoring multiple sites at any given time to act as a support to the onsite team, which has hands-on control to change the course of events. Like an air traffic controller, the eNurse or ePhysician monitors the situation with a broad view and has access to various additional forms of information that are not always readily available to onsite team members. The eTeam, like the air traffic controller, is instantaneously accessible to gather and relay information that is requested from the onsite team. Its members can also actively offer recommendations for actions to be taken by the onsite team members, whether they are pilots or medical professionals, to ensure a safer and higher-quality outcome. In air traffic control and the eICU model of care, effective communication and interactions between those at the remote control center and onsite are critical to the success of the practice model.

The essence of working in the eICU work environment is the supportive team environment that has been created for the sole purpose of supporting the bedside clinicians with experienced ICU nurses and intensivists to provide the best possible care to ICU patients. Interactions with the bedside team are either passive or active. In the passive mode, the eTeam is readily available when contacted by the bedside team. In the active mode, the eTeam has identified a need for a patient intervention and it contacts the bedside team to take action. The irony is that the bedside team is often skeptical, not appreciative and offended by the active mode of support. For the ICU patient care team to become integral and contributing members of the team, the eClinicians must constantly practice collaborative communication in order not to offend the bedside health care workers.

Across the board, the eNurses very much enjoy the eICU work environment. They see it as a way to continue to use their critical thinking skills and years of ICU experience in a setting with less physical demands than bedside ICU nursing. Although all of the ePhysicians interviewed saw value in the eICU model of care from a patient safety and cost-avoidance perspective, most were quick to point out that the ideal situation is to have an intensivist physically present in the ICU. eNurses and ePhysicians recognize that experienced ICU nurses and intensivists are in limited supply. They believe the eICU model of care is a viable way to stretch those limited resources over a broad number of ICU patients by using a telemedicine platform.

Further study is needed to describe the view and effectiveness of the eICU model of care from the perspective of the bedside ICU team. This perspective is needed to determine how to develop appropriate protocols, policies, communication plans, and practices that will ensure ongoing effective collaboration between the two entities.

REFERENCES

1. Kowalczyk L. Tele-treatment. 2007. Available at: http://www.boston.com/business/globe/articles/2007/11/19/tele_treatment/?page=1. Accessed on May 30, 2008.
2. International Society for Telemedicine & eHealth. 2008. Available at: http://www.isft.net/cms/index.php?aid=21. Accessed May 30, 2008.

3. Rosenfeld BA, Dorman T, Breslow MJ, et al. Intensive care unit telemedicine: alternate paradigm for providing continuous intensivist care. Crit Care Med 2000;28(12):3925–31.

4. Becker C. Remote control: specialists are running intensive-care units from remote sites via computers, and at least one health system with the e-ICU is reaping financial rewards and saving lives. Mod Healthc 2002;32:40–2.

5. Breslow MJ, Rosenfeld BA, Doerfler M, et al. Effect of a multiple-site intensive care unit telemedicine program on clinical and economic outcomes: an alternative paradigm for intensivist staffing. Crit Care Med 2004;32(1):31–8.

6. Blumer H. Symbolic interactionism: perspective and method. Englewood Cliffs (NJ): Prentice-Hall; 1969.

7. Charon JM. Symbolic interactionism: an introduction, an interpretation, an integration. 9th edition. Upper Saddle River (NJ): Prentice Hall; 2007.

8. Hoey BA (n.d.). What is ethnography?. Available at: http://www.brianhoey.com/General%20Site/general_defn-ethnography.htm. Accessed June 30, 2007.

9. Kotarba JA, Hurt D. An ethnography of an AIDS hospice: toward a theory of organizational pastiche. Symbolic Interaction 1995;18(4):413–38.

10. Borbasi S, Jackson D, Wilkes L. Fieldwork in nursing research: positionality, practicalities, and predicaments. J Adv Nurs 2003;51(5):493–501.

11. Buller S, Butterworth T. Skilled nursing practice: a qualitative study of the elements of nursing. Int J Nurs Stud 2000;38:405–17.

12. Lincoln YS, Guba EG. Naturalistic inquiry. Beverly Hills (CA): Sage Publications, Inc; 1985.

13. Lofland J, Lofland J. Analyzing social settings: a guide to qualitative observation and analysis. 3rd edition. Belmont (CA): Wadsworth; 1995.

14. VISICU. eICU® care delivery. Available at: http://www.visicu.com/products/services/clinicalservices.html. Accessed on June 25, 2008.

A Patient- and Family-Centered Care Model Paves the Way for a Culture of Quality and Safety

Patricia Reid Ponte, RN, DNSc, FAAN[a,b,*],
Kenneth Peterson, MS, MA, RN[c,d]

KEYWORDS

- Quality • Safety • Patient- and family-centered care

Innovative care delivery models are now among the key drivers for improving quality in health care. A model of care delivery is composed of multiple structural and process elements, including an organized framework for interactions and decision making; a prescribed set of work flow processes; providers, care givers, support staff, patients, and families, each with clearly defined roles and authority; and goals or outputs that are most often described in terms of specific clinical, practice, service, and process outcomes.[1] The extent to which a care delivery model can improve performance and service effectiveness (ie, care quality and patient safety) depends on its relationship to the organizational culture and whether the model and culture are driven by the same values and goals.

Over the past decade, a growing number of organizations, including the Institute of Medicine, the Agency for Healthcare Research and Quality, and The Joint Commission, have called on organizations to adopt more patient-centered models of care.[2–5] In such models, providers and clinicians partner with patients and families throughout the course of treatment, and the perspectives of patients and families influence the design of care processes and organizational decision making.

Dana-Farber Cancer Institute (DFCI) is one of many organizations that have acted on the recommendations of these groups. DFCI's move toward a patient- and family-centered model of care was prompted in part by its decision to form a joint clinical partnership with Brigham and Women's Hospital (BWH) in 1995. To assure that patient needs would drive decision making and care delivery processes affected by the partnership, DFCI's leaders and patients and families began examining the principles that underlie patient- and family-centered care and took steps to incorporate them into organizational planning and patient care practices. DFCI's commitment to patient- and family-centered care was reinforced by the learning that occurred following two tragic medication errors, which highlighted the importance of listening to and partnering with patients and families. As the patient- and family-centered care model took root, DFCI leaders, providers, and staff realized that tapping into the diverse perspectives, knowledge, and passions of patients and families not only bolstered the organization's efforts to

[a] Nursing and Patient Care Services, Dana-Farber Cancer Institute, Boston, MA, USA
[b] Oncology Nursing and Clinical Services, Brigham and Women's Hospital, Boston, MA, USA
[c] Plumley Village Health Services, University of Massachusetts Memorial Medical Center, Worcester, MA, USA
[d] The Heller School for Social Policy and Management, Brandeis University, Waltham, MA, USA
* Corresponding author. Nursing and Patient Care Services, Dana-Farber Cancer Institute, 44 Binney Street, Boston, MA 02114.
E-mail address: Pat_reid_ponte@dfci.harvard.edu (P. Reid Ponte).

Crit Care Nurs Clin N Am 20 (2008) 451–464
doi:10.1016/j.ccell.2008.08.001

achieve excellence in care and clinical trials but also added significantly to the quality, safety, operational effectiveness, and long-term strategic direction of organizational structures, processes, and outcomes.

In this article, the authors describe how DFCI designed, implemented, and advanced a patient- and family-centered care delivery model that shaped the evolution of the practice environment, governance structures, and work processes, and contributed to the creation of a culture of quality and safety. The authors also discuss key organizational commitments and structures that underpin the model, and the quality and safety efforts at DFCI.

DIMENSIONS OF PATIENT- AND FAMILY-CENTERED CARE

Patient-centered care delivery models have been prominent in the health care literature for many years. These models are based on the perspective that patients should be at the center of the care delivery process and are distinctly different from models emphasizing illness, diagnostic, provider, or system-centered approaches to care.[2,6–11] In recent years, the term "patient-centered care" has been expanded to "patient- and family-centered care," highlighting the role that families play in the care of patients, and their contributions to a patient's overall health and well-being.[11]

Definitions for patient-centered and patient- and family-centered care range from simple descriptions to multidimensional frameworks. One simple definition describes patient-centered care as understanding the patient as a unique human being.[12] Other definitions describe it as a style of consulting in which the doctor uses the patient's knowledge to guide the interaction,[13] and as viewing the patient's illness through the patient's own eyes.[14]

In the early 1990s, the Picker/Commonwealth Program for Patient Centered Care completed a seminal piece of work in which it examined patients' needs and concerns through patient focus groups and surveys and used the results to identify the following seven dimensions of patient-centered care: respect for patients' values, preferences, and expressed needs; coordination and integration of care; information, communication, and education; physical comfort; emotional support and alleviation of fear and anxiety; involvement of family and friends; and transition and continuity.[7] The group later added access to reliable care as an eighth dimension.[15]

Over the years, the Picker/Commonwealth view of patient-centered care has become the most widely recognized model for individualized care delivery in the health care arena. Since it was proposed, some investigators have expanded on it to emphasize the importance of sharing information and involving patients in decision making,[16] and of assuring that the care that is delivered is congruent with, and responsive to, a patient's wants, needs, and preferences.[17]

The Institute for Family-Centered Care, a group dedicated to advancing the understanding and practice of patient- and family-centered care, identifies four core concepts of patient- and family-centered care: dignity and respect, information sharing, participation, and collaboration. The institute notes that these concepts should not only guide interactions between patients and providers at the individual level but also should form the basis of the relationship between patients and families and the organization as a whole. Health care institutions, it suggests, should involve patients and families in activities related to policy and program development, health care facility design, and professional education.[18,19] Several organizations have responded to this suggestion by creating patient and family advisory councils (PFACs) and other internal mechanisms to assure that patients and families are involved in decision making at the institutional and unit level.[20–23]

As organizations gain experience with patient- and family-centered care, many have come to realize that developing a relationship with patients and families and involving them in their own care contributes to quality care and patient safety.[9,24,25] As a result, several prominent oversight groups have started urging health care organizations to adopt patient-centered care as a safety strategy. In their 2001 landmark report, *Crossing the Quality Chasm*, the Institute of Medicine urged the adoption of patient-centered care as one of six aims for improving the safety of the health care system.[2] Similarly, The Joint Commission began requiring hospitals to encourage patients' active involvement in their own care as part of its 2008 National Patient Safety Goals.[5]

CORE ELEMENTS OF A CULTURE OF QUALITY AND SAFETY

Interest in patient-centered care as a safety strategy reflects a growing awareness among health care providers of quality and safety issues affecting care delivery, including those stemming from errors, waste, and the overuse or underuse of various treatments and care practices. The number of deaths due to iatrogenic injury and illness, adverse drug events, or other errors has been estimated to be as high as 44,000 to

98,000 per year.[26] These numbers, however, tell just part of the story. Wasteful practices related to billing, duplicate history taking, missing records, delays, and poor access account for other quality and safety gaps.[27] Additional problems stem from the overuse of procedures and the overprescribing of medications, while still others occur as a result of the underuse of therapies shown to be effective, such as some vaccines, screening practices, and medications such as post–myocardial infarction beta blockers.[28,29]

Over the past decade, many health care institutions have redesigned their quality programs and launched new initiatives to eliminate unsafe practices and improve patient safety. In many of these organizations, assuring safe, high-quality patient care has become a motivating force for leaders, providers, and staff and a culture of quality and safety focused on minimizing hazards and patient harm[30] has taken root.

As noted by Ken Kizer, MD, past president of the National Quality Forum, cultures of quality and safety are characterized by the following five critical elements:[31]

A Commitment to Continuous Learning and Process Redesign

Organizations that are committed to improving patient safety are open to new ideas, seek out best practices, and continually work to identify and address quality and safety gaps. Leaders in these organizations realize they must nurture a propensity for listening to patients, families, staff, and providers, and treat any concerns and complaints that are expressed as opportunities for improvement. They must also encourage staff and other leaders to review and replicate best practices and engage in research and improvement efforts that help them identify better ways of doing things.

A System for Error Identification, Mitigation, and Evaluation

Having methods to identify flawed systems and practices is critical for successful patient safety efforts. Methods that can be used include human factors analysis, safety rounds, and early detection and prevention strategies. Using technology and other mechanisms to reduce variation and errors is also critical. These mechanisms include clinical practice guidelines, decision support systems, and technologies that support medication order entry and longitudinal medical records.

A Process to Assure Clinical/Technical, Interpersonal, and Analytic Competence in Quality Management and Care Planning and Delivery Practices

Providers, clinicians, and staff must be as skilled in quality improvement practices as they are in care planning and delivery. The competency model for each group should be explicitly based on the values of the organization and should highlight the required clinical and technical skills and knowledge and the behavioral expectations related to teamwork, leadership, diversity, respect, patient- and family-centered care, confidentiality, quality management, process improvement, and ethics. The competency model must be supplemented by a commitment from managers to develop and manage performance goals at the individual level, monitor compliance, and assure employee access to appropriate education and training activities. By actively managing clinicians and other staff, managers ensure that all members of the organization receive the preparation, guidance, and support they need to practice safely and consistently and contribute to quality and safety goals.

An Organization-Wide Methodology for Establishing Priorities, Developing Goals and Objectives, and Managing Performance

Management reporting systems, such as dashboards and scorecards, provide information that allows leaders, providers, and staff throughout the organization to establish improvement goals and to benchmark the progress of improvement initiatives. These systems should cascade up and down the organization so that all members of the organization, from patients and families to members of the board, have a clear understanding of the institution's performance related to quality and safety.

Interdisciplinary Collaboration and Teamwork as the Norm

Creating a culture of safety requires ongoing interdisciplinary collaboration and the commitment of every discipline and department. Such collaboration is more apt to occur when the organization maintains an interdisciplinary leadership model in which nurses, physicians, and administrators have equal and complementary roles as leaders of major clinical programs and initiatives. Such a leadership model creates a climate in which all providers and staff view one another as internal customers and respect members of other departments and disciplines for their unique insights and contributions. An interdisciplinary leadership structure also provides an effective framework for assuring that care is highly coordinated and anticipates patient and family needs, a place where the culture of quality and safety and patient- and family-centered care intersect.

Organizations committed to quality and safety and patient- and family-centered care view both areas as major priorities and constantly work on assuring their continued evolution. Leaders in these organizations "walk the talk" by involving front-line staff, providers, and patients and families in planning and implementing organizational priorities and they consistently demonstrate and insist on respectful behavior by all staff, clinicians, and providers. They also assure that organizational systems are designed to enhance patient safety and quality and to support interdisciplinary practice and patient care across the continuum.

PATIENT- AND FAMILY-CENTERED CARE AND QUALITY AND SAFETY AT DANA-FARBER CANCER INSTITUTE

DFCI's commitment to a patient- and family-centered model of care was prompted by its decision to enter into a joint clinical partnership with BWH in 1995. Through the joint partnership, inpatient medical oncology services would move from DFCI to BWH, and medical oncology ambulatory services would move from BWH to DFCI. As DFCI's interdisciplinary executive leadership team considered this major organizational change, it began asking important questions about how the two organizations could assure that the needs of patients and families would drive decision making and that patients and families would be positioned at the center of care and clinical trials. At the same time, several patients who were highly invested in DFCI's future stepped forward to express their concerns about the partnership and its potential impact on patient care. In short, they wanted assurance that patients and families would be at the center of, and central to, care processes that were developed as a result of the joint venture and they asked to be involved in planning this major organizational change.

This coming together of resolute patients with interdisciplinary leaders who believed in the centrality of patients and families resulted in a series of meetings in which both groups explored the role patients and families might play in influencing and providing direction for the joint clinical partnership. Working together, institutional leaders and patients and families identified ways to involve patients and family members in merging operations at the two organizations. As DFCI leaders witnessed the value that patients and

families brought to this effort, they decided to expand how patients and families were involved in DFCI's activities by creating two PFACs (one for adult care and one for pediatrics). Over time, these councils have become integral to DFCI's strategic planning and decision-making processes, and to the joint clinical programs that DFCI maintains with its partnering institutions (ie, Dana-Farber/Brigham and Women's Cancer Center [DF/BWCC] and Dana-Farber/Children's Hospital Cancer Center). Through monthly meetings, council members provide input into organizational policies and decisions. They also serve on a wide array of committees and improvement teams at the unit and organizational level and play a pivotal role in assuring quality and safety at DFCI. The Chief Nursing Officer (CNO), the Chief Medical Officer (CMO), and the Chief Operating Officer (COO) are members of the councils and are routinely present at the monthly council meetings.[20]

Another factor that contributed to DFCI's decision to move toward a patient- and family-centered model of care was the occurrence of two medication errors involving chemotherapy overdoses that led to the death of one patient and the serious injury of another. These events, which have been described in detail in other publications,[32,33] led to a period of deep reflection within the organization and a comprehensive examination of patient care systems and practices. By reviewing the days and events that led to the patient's death, DFCI leaders, providers, and staff came to realize that the patient knew something was not right during the hours before she died and tried to communicate this to her care team. At that time, however, viewing the patient as a partner in care, and as someone who possesses information and knowledge that should be added to the care plan, was not central to DFCI's care model. As a result, the patient's concerns were not recognized as information that might be used to guide clinical care planning. Witnessing the consequences of this and of many system-level flaws served as a wake-up call for every person in the organization and galvanized DFCI's commitment to patient- and family-centered care and to patient safety and quality.

BUILDING A CULTURE OF QUALITY AND SAFETY

Quality and safety have always been top priorities at DFCI; however, work to develop a culture of quality and safety escalated markedly over the last decade, simultaneous with a surge in patient volume and clinical trial activity. Shortly after the chemotherapy overdoses occurred, the organization launched a series of initiatives focused on improving the systems that support medication administration. Some of the programs, initiatives, and innovations introduced were based on best practices recommended by other organizations, whereas others reflected the original insights and ideas of DFCI leaders, providers, and staff. At the same time, DFCI leaders introduced changes in the organizational structure to assure strong interdisciplinary clinical practice and to engage the board of trustees in the patient safety and patient- and family-centered care efforts. (This work is documented in an article by Conway and colleagues[34] describing our "10-year journey" and many of the lessons learned.)

Clinicians at DFCI also began working to develop a set of robust information technology systems, including a longitudinal medical record system and a state-of-the-art chemotherapy order entry system designed to standardize orders based on templates, to detect errors and inconsistencies, and to eliminate many of the problems that occur with paper-based systems. The work to develop these systems was accompanied by a renewed commitment to proactive risk assessment and error mitigation and the introduction of error response practices that encourage nonpunitive reporting and the routine use of root cause analysis.

DFCI's work to create a safer care environment ultimately involved every leader, provider, and member of the cancer center staff. Improving patient quality and safety became the focus of the board, the executive leadership team, and improvement teams at the program and unit levels. Through this level of involvement, a culture of quality and safety took root that continues to advance to this day.

THE IMPORTANCE OF PARTNERSHIP

Collaboration and partnering with patients and families, and with one another, underlies DFCI's approach to care, service, quality, and research, and was central to our efforts to adopt a patient- and family-centered model of care and a culture of quality and safety. DFCI's commitment to partnering is evidenced by the collaborative relationships it enjoys with many other health care organizations and providers, including the joint clinical partnership with BWH described earlier and a similar partnership with Children's Hospital Boston dedicated to providing pediatric oncology care. Partnership is also at the core of the Dana-Farber Harvard Cancer Center (DFHCC), one of 46 comprehensive cancer centers recognized by the National Cancer Institute. Through DFHCC, DFCI collaborates with six other institutions

(BWH, Children's Hospital Boston, Beth Israel Deaconess Medical Center, Massachusetts General Hospital, Harvard Medical School, and the Harvard School of Public Health) to coordinate cancer research efforts and promote collaboration among cancer scientists. In addition, DFCI partners with Massachusetts General Hospital and other organizations that are part of Partners Health Care, a large integrated health system in the area, to assure positive competition and alignment of resources, and overall service quality and coordination of oncology services.

The need to partner well in all realms has had a strong influence on DFCI's organizational culture and has facilitated the development and implementation of an interdisciplinary leadership and governance model. In this model, leadership triads composed of a nurse, physician, and administrator are responsible for clinical operations and decision making at the organization and program levels. Other disciplines critical to oncology care, such as pharmacists, social workers, nutritionists, and other allied health staff are also central to this governance model. (More information about the leadership model is shared below.) The model assures that all disciplines are engaged in priority setting and quality monitoring and improvement activities and, as a result, it has become the foundation for DFCI's culture of safety. It also assures an interdisciplinary approach and commitment to patient- and family-centered care.

ADVANCING A CULTURE OF QUALITY AND SAFETY AND PATIENT- AND FAMILY-CENTERED CARE: REQUIRED ORGANIZATIONAL COMMITMENTS

DFCI's experience highlights key values, structures, and processes that organizations must introduce and maintain to advance a patient- and family-centered model of care and a culture of quality and safety. These required commitments include the following:

Interdisciplinary Leadership Through a Nurse-Physician-Administrative Leadership Model

Many academic medical centers still maintain a hierarchic leadership structure. Although such a structure may allow them to operate extremely well at the department level, it often complicates efforts to work across disciplines and departments. A hierarchic structure can also result in less than optimal planning and decision making at the organization and unit levels and can lead to power struggles that compromise patient care, research, and other activities that require a cross-functional approach.

To avoid the problems associated with a hierarchic model, DFCI implemented a collaborative leadership model in which leadership triads composed of a nurse, physician, and administrator are responsible for clinical operations and decision making at the organization and program levels. This collaborative and integrated structure eliminates the phenomenon of having one discipline or department try to avoid or handicap change and assures that the work of planning, organizing, and implementing integrated patient care processes is executed successfully. However, the effective use of this leadership model does not come naturally or easily. Among the methods used to facilitate the model and assure its success are collaborative practice agreements through which the triad members agree to collaborate with one another and commit to working through disagreements.[35,36] The leaders must also work together to develop a strategy for communicating with each other and with staff and to decide who will take the lead on particular projects and programs.

DFCI's executive leadership triad is composed of the CMO, COO, and CNO. (As the senior vice president of Patient Care Services, the CNO has accountability for nursing and for the disciplines of social work, care coordination, pharmacy, nutrition, and other allied health programs). Working together, this group oversees operations at the organizational level and is responsible for program approval and resource and policy decisions that require executive input. The executive triad also leads various quality and safety initiatives and programs and uses these to foster the involvement of front-line staff and assure that clinicians and staff help drive priorities and change. One recent project focused on improving patient flow. For this project, all three members of the triad served as project leaders and were responsible for initiating major decisions and driving the work of the project team.

The members of the executive triad also chair many committees that cross institutional lines. For example, the CNO chairs the DF/BWCC Quality Committee, the CMO chairs the DF/BWCC Service Line Committee, and the COO chairs the DF/BW Executive Leadership Group. In all cases, the person serving as the committee chair acknowledges the other triad members and assures that each of them agrees on the committee's decisions and priorities. Gaining such agreement takes discipline, exquisite communication and collaboration, and attentiveness to conflict management and resolution, which are achieved through weekly meetings; frequent e-mail communications, clarifications, and deliberations; and quarterly extended work sessions. In some cases, the triad seeks additional input from the chief executive officer (CEO), department chairs, and other members of senior leadership. Any disagreements among the triad members are worked out before a final decision is communicated to the committees. Similar interdisciplinary leadership triads at the director and managerial levels oversee the clinical programs and services within DFCI and observe the same practices related to collaboration, communication, and decision making.

Patient and Family Involvement in Organizational Decision Making

Partnering with patients and families to provide direct care and to plan organizational strategy, policies, and initiatives is no small feat. The principles of partnership, transparency, and information sharing must guide interactions between providers and patients and families at the bedside and be applied to decision making at the organizational level. To include patients and families in organizational decision making, systems and structures must be modified to ensure that patients and families have a voice in planning organizational strategy and in designing changes and improvements in patient care and clinical services. A disciplined approach must be used to ensure that no major decisions related to clinical services are made without questioning whether the patient and family perspective would benefit planning, implementation, and evaluation efforts.

At DFCI, the PFACs provide the infrastructure to support this important work.[20] (See adult PFAC bylaws, Appendix 1.) The adult and pediatric PFACs are composed of volunteer patients and family members and meet monthly to organize the work of their members. The work takes many different forms and includes participating on institutional councils, committees, and work teams; on search committees for senior executives and nurse managers; and on unit-based practice committees and program development task forces. In addition, one member of each council sits on DFCI's Joint Quality Improvement and Risk Management Committee, a board-level committee that is composed of members of the board of trustees and senior members of the organization, and that is charged with reviewing DFCI's annual quality improvement plan, ongoing improvement activities, and sentinel event reports.

One interesting side effect of having patients and families involved in decision making is that group leaders are now more apt to ensure that others who can provide useful insights are also involved. When group leaders ask, "Is a PFAC member present?" or, "Should the PFAC be involved in this planning and decision making?" another question inevitably follows (ie, "Should one of our front-line staff or providers be present for this decision?") As a result, many decisions are informed by diverse perspectives, and individuals throughout the organization help drive organizational strategy and operations.

Transparency and Openness by Executive Leadership

Organizations can foster openness and transparency by regularly bringing leaders and staff together and encouraging them to share their perspectives with one another. At DFCI, several different processes have been designed to foster discussion among leaders and staff representing diverse roles, disciplines, and perspectives. Using such a cross-functional approach results in considerable give-and-take and often yields powerful new insights.

One mechanism used to foster interaction among leaders, providers, and staff is the President's Forum. During this 2-hour session, 25 to 30 leaders and staff interact with one another and with a panel composed of the CEO, CNO, CFO, COO, chief information officer, and chief scientific officer. Participants pose questions to the panel and panel members respond extemporaneously, one person taking the lead and the others joining in, depending on the issue being addressed. Another forum that encourages interaction between leaders and staff is called "Breakfast with Pat," in which the CNO, and often one of her direct reports, join 8 to 10 staff from different disciplines for a 1-hour, early morning breakfast session. The CNO engages in an informal discussion with attendees, asking why they chose to work at DFCI, querying them about challenges they have encountered, and sharing information about current organizational priorities and initiatives. Yet another forum is Patient Safety Rounds, in which the CNO, CMO, or COO (or all three), along with the vice presidents for safety and quality and a member of the board of trustees, go to a unit or practice area and interact with the interdisciplinary team of clinicians and support staff. During these sessions, they ask participants to share their safety and quality concerns and to describe problems that concern them. The issues that are raised tend to be practice oriented, practical, and specific. Because the rounds are conducted on the unit, they give senior leaders and board members a better appreciation of how

the issues impact providers, staff, patients, and families.

These forums, which encourage open dialog among executive leaders and staff, have become central to our culture of quality and safety. Keeping the sessions informal, by not planning the agendas in advance and keeping interactions among the executive team and staff unchoreographed, encourages participants to engage in a dialog with leaders and to share their safety concerns and insights and suggestions for improvement.

A Fair and Just Culture and Systems for Error Identification and Mitigation

To improve patient safety, organizations must be able to detect and address readily problems and factors that contribute to system failures. One of the most effective ways to identify such factors is by reviewing and investigating errors that are reported by staff. Developing a culture in which staff are not afraid to report errors and near-misses is extremely challenging because in many organizations, a lingering propensity exists to respond to mistakes in a way that is the social norm (ie, to blame someone).

Moving from a culture of blame to one that embraces nonpunitive reporting and that is guided by the principles of fairness and justice is hard work and demands the commitment of leaders at every level. It also requires creating an environment that allows staff to "raise their hands" and report errors without the fear of retribution. Reporting an error or near-miss should launch a process that focuses not on individual misdeeds, but on exploring and uncovering the system failures that are contributing factors.

In the years after the chemotherapy overdoses, DFCI started using root cause analysis and similar techniques to examine problems and identify systemic factors that contributed to errors. This process helped us appreciate the value of responding to errors and near-misses with a consistent and nonpunitive approach, and led us to develop a set of "Principles of a Fair and Just Culture" (Appendix 2) to guide the actions of leaders and staff and encourage error reporting.[37] These principles reflect the understanding that although problems with individual accountability may occasionally contribute to errors and must be addressed, most errors occur as a result of inadequate and problematic systems. We have learned that the best way to prevent errors is to develop a climate that encourages individuals to identify errors and near-misses, and that promotes open discussion, learning, and shared problem solving. We have also learned that executives, managers, and staff are more likely to adopt a non-punitive approach when tools, such as the Principles of a Fair and Just Culture, guidelines for error reporting and investigation, and sample case studies are developed, disseminated, and revisited frequently over time.

Respectful Interdisciplinary Collaboration and Team Effectiveness

Interdisciplinary collaboration and teamwork are critical to advancing patient- and family-centered care and patient safety. Helping leaders, providers, and staff learn to collaborate effectively can be difficult, however, particularly when traditions and norms based on hierarchy still linger in the organization and one believes that power starts and stays at the top. One industry that offers a model for helping employees acquire these skills is the airline industry, which over the last 2 decades has undergone transformational change marked by the creation of policies and the use of team approaches that resulted in enhanced cockpit crew effectiveness and airline safety.[38,39]

Although respectful interdisciplinary collaboration is now part of the DFCI culture, maintaining and continuing to foster such collaboration requires the ongoing attention of senior leaders. The CEO has taken the lead in this area by telling his senior leaders to have zero tolerance for any disrespectful behaviors and attitudes and by becoming directly involved in addressing difficult behaviors encountered among senior leaders, providers, and staff. We have used several other strategies to continuously promote respectful interdisciplinary collaboration. These strategies include a "respect retreat" that was attended by all providers and staff at the midmanager and senior director levels. The CEO opened the retreat and set the stage for the 4-hour session, which used a workshop approach and case studies to stimulate discussion. We have also begun to provide team effectiveness training and are considering developing a compact or credo describing behavior standards, which would be signed by all providers and staff.

Magnet Program of Nursing Excellence

The Magnet Recognition Program developed by the American Nurses Credentialing Center and the American Academy of Nursing provides a blueprint for achieving excellence in nursing practice and patient care. The new Magnet model is composed of five key elements: transformational leadership; structured empowerment; exemplary professional nursing practice; new knowledge, innovations, and improvements; and empiric quality outcomes.[40] Each of these elements contains factors, or "forces of magnetism," that are critical for developing and retaining a high-quality nursing workforce.[41,42] Studies have shown that practice environments that embody these factors are associated with better patient outcomes.[43–46]

DFCI attained Magnet designation in 2005. Our work to achieve this designation involved the efforts of providers and staff throughout the organization and resulted in the creation of an extraordinary practice environment and a positive and enduring culture of excellence. Like other worthwhile endeavors, the process of assuring that the 14 Forces of Magnetism are present and enculturated into practice required the leadership, hard work, and dedication of leaders and staff throughout the organization; however, the benefits resulting from this work are many. In addition to achieving Magnet recognition, we believe we also raised our level of nursing practice and enhanced the quality of care and patient safety throughout the institution.

Based on our experience, we recommend that hospitals striving to achieve excellence in quality and safety embark on the journey to attain Magnet designation. Just as the work to create a culture of quality and safety is never over, the Magnet journey is also never finished because it inspires leaders and staff in the organization to strive continuously for higher levels of excellence.

Evidence-Based Practice, Clinical Effectiveness, and Continuous Learning

By generating new knowledge and developing and testing new approaches to care, organizations not only achieve clinical effectiveness but also lay the groundwork for evidence-based practice and high-quality care. At DFCI, a longstanding commitment to discovery and impact underlies our support for research in the basic sciences, clinical effectiveness, quality of life, health services, psychosocial oncology, and integrative therapies. By supporting research in these areas, we are creating the knowledge base necessary for evidence-based practice, quality improvement, and organizational change, and are helping to "decrease the burden of cancer," a goal central to DFCI's mission.

Nursing's commitment to continued discovery is evidenced by a robust Center for Nursing and Patient Care Services Research. The center is dedicated to expanding clinical science and evidence-based practice in oncology nursing. In addition to conducting their own research, the center's nurse-scientists work with staff nurses to identify best practices in cancer care. The center's current projects include a study focused on improving adherence to oral chemotherapy regimens, and a study examining the use of intravenous lines in the pediatric oncology clinic. The results of these and other projects are disseminated and relevant findings are incorporated into care policies.

Systems Thinking, Process Improvement, and Clinical Quality Improvement Framework

Improving patient care and safety requires a deep understanding of systems thinking and an infrastructure for ongoing quality monitoring and management and process improvement. Developing such capabilities is especially important in today's organizations, which face constant pressure to expand and to adopt an ever-growing array of treatments and technologies.

At DFCI, our approach to clinical quality management has been shaped by our involvement in the National Comprehensive Cancer Network (NCCN) and its efforts to develop, implement, and evaluate clinical guidelines. (The NCCN is an alliance composed of 21 of the world's leading cancer centers.)[47] In contrast, developing a process improvement methodology for the organization, including approaches for increasing efficiency and decreasing waste, has only recently become a priority. Several factors, including the rapid growth of services on DFCI's main campus and the expansion of our distributed campus and network practices, have highlighted the need for such a methodology. Through our work in the area of patient safety, our managers, providers, and staff have developed a sound understanding of systems thinking; however, they now need to develop a more solid footing in quality monitoring techniques and in methods to improve and assure the standardization of processes across practice settings. A work team led by the COO, CNO, CMO, the vice president of quality and risk management, and the vice president of the Center for Patient Safety are currently examining organizational needs in this area and are developing an organization-wide framework to assure a disciplined approach to annual priority setting, project approval and management, and the appropriate use of process improvement and clinical quality techniques.

SUMMARY

DFCI has undergone continual and positive change over the last decade. This change has been steeped in our commitment to patient- and family-centered care and to building a culture of quality and safety. The organization's tradition of partnering has formed the basis for all of our efforts. We have learned that to partner effectively, each party must remain open and committed to learning from one another. The knowledge and insight we have gained through our partnerships with patients and families, other organizations, and with one another have allowed us to improve continually the quality and safety of the care we provide, and have helped us create a patient- and family-centered practice environment in which staff, providers, and leaders thrive.

ACKNOWLEDGMENTS

The authors thank Beth Kantz, RN, and Jane Corrigan Wandel, RN, of Corrigan Kantz Consulting for editing support.

APPENDIX 1: DANA-FARBER/BRIGHAM AND WOMEN'S CANCER CENTER ADULT PATIENT AND FAMILY ADVISORY COUNCIL BYLAWS
Article I. Name

The name of the organization is Adult Patient and Family Advisory Council of the Dana-Farber/Brigham and Women's Cancer Center. It is sometimes referred to as the APFAC. It is also called the Council.

Article II. Mission

The Adult Patient and Family Advisory Council is dedicated to assuring the delivery of the highest standards of comprehensive and compassionate health care by Dana-Farber/Brigham and Women's Cancer Center. We do this by working in active partnership with our health care providers to:

> Strengthen communication and collaboration among patients, families, caregivers and staff
>
> Promote patient and family advocacy and involvement
>
> Propose and participate in oncology programs, services, and policies

Article III. Members

Section 1. Membership Eligibility. Patients, family members, and staff from the Dana-Farber/Brigham and Women's Cancer Center are eligible to be members of the Council. Members should be committed to building a partnership of advisors and staff working to understand the needs of the constituents they represent and to implement programs and policies to address health care challenges within the participating institutions.

Section 2. Council Makeup. The Council's voting membership will be made up of a broad base of up to 17 patients and/or family active members (at least two-thirds patients) and up to 5 staff members from the main DF/BWCC campus in the Longwood Medical Area.

Section 3. Participation. Members are expected to participate in monthly meetings consisting of 2–3 hours and in various committees or projects that will require a varied number of hours. They will be required to participate on a minimum of one committee or project at all times.

Section 4. Active Membership. A term of Active Membership consists of one year, renewable each year for a maximum of 3 terms. Individuals will be polled for their preference for continued membership at the end of each year. All Active members must be in compliance with the requirements for active volunteer status.

Section 5. Vacancies/Leaves of Absence. Council members may resign or request a leave of absence from the Council at any time during their term. A member may request a leave of absence when unusual or unavoidable circumstances require that the member be absent from meetings and activities for an extended period, up to one year. The member will submit his/her request in writing to the co-chairs, stating the reason for the request and the length of time requested. The co-chairs will determine if the request will be accepted. If a member cannot return at the end of the requested leave, he/she will resign from the Council. At any resignation, the Council may choose to add a replacement at that time or to leave the position open until the next rotation of members.

Section 6. Recruitment. Council members and the Institutions' staff will be utilized to recruit and recommend future members.

Section 7. Selection. Potential members will fill out a volunteer application form. The Council's program manager will consult with the director of Volunteer Services and then will conduct a phone interview. After successful completion of the interview the candidate will be invited to a Council meeting. One or two of the co-chairs will interview the potential member for one-half hour before the monthly meeting. The co-chairs, with consideration of comments from the Council and staff, will determine the candidate's eligibility for membership. The program manager will notify the potential member of the decision.

Section 8. Emeritus Members. Council members who have served three terms may become Emeritus Members. They will be welcome at all Council meetings and will continue to represent the council on committees and projects if their volunteer status is current and active. They will not have Council voting privileges.

Section 9. Associate Members. Approved candidates for membership will become Associate Members if there is not an open position on the Council at the time of approval. Associate members will be welcome at Council meetings. They will not have Council voting privileges but they may represent the Council on committees and projects if their volunteer status is current and active. They will remain Associate Members until a patient or family member position on the Council becomes available.

Section 10. Alumni/ae Status. Those Council members who would be eligible for Emeritus membership but no longer can attend Council meetings and participate on committees or projects (no longer can fulfill the role of an Emeritus member) will be named Alumni/ae. They will have the option to remain on the Council's email distribution list. Alumni/ae members will not have Council voting privileges, nor will they attend Council meetings or participate on committees or projects. They will not be required to maintain volunteer compliance.

Article IV. DF/BWCC Satellite Representation

Section 1. Participation. The Council shall welcome participation from patients, family members, and staff from each DF/BWCC satellite location.

Article V. Officers

Section 1. Officers and Duties. There shall be two chairpersons, known as Co-chairs. The Co-chairs will be responsible for setting Council meeting agendas, chairing and conducting meetings, coordinating between Council members and staff, providing leadership for the Council members and serving on Institutions' committees where the Chairs are specifically requested.

Section 2. Nomination Procedure. Candidates for the co-chair position will be nominated from Council members having at least one year of experience as a Council member. A nominating committee may be selected by the Council. Nominations will also be accepted from the floor prior to election.

Section 3. Election Procedure. Officers will be elected by the affirmative vote of two-thirds of the members present and voting.

Section 4. Term. The standard term will be two years, even if this means the co-chair will serve 4, one-year active membership terms. The term of office will begin the January 1st after the office is elected, unless otherwise specified.

Section 5. Vacancies. A Co-Chair may resign from office at any time. The Council may choose to elect a replacement to complete the term of the officer or to leave the position open until the next scheduled election.

Article VI. Meetings

Section 1. Regular Meetings. Regular meetings of the Adult Patient and Family Advisory Council will be held on the second Tuesday of each month from 5:30 PM to 8:00 PM unless otherwise ordered, presuming the presence of a quorum.

Section 2. Special Meetings. Special meetings may be called by the Council Co-chairs as they deem necessary. Council members will be given at least 24 hours notice of the meeting schedule and agenda.

Section 3. Quorum. An official meeting will require the presence of a minimum of one-half of the members to be called to order.

Section 4. Voting. Votes may be conducted electronically for most items, except where specifically requested to be in person. Electronic votes will require a response (yes, no, or abstain) from a quorum of members.

Article VII. Amendment Procedure

These bylaws may be amended at any regular meeting of the Council by the affirmative vote of two-thirds of the members present and voting, provided that the amendment has been submitted in writing at the previous regular meeting.

APPENDIX 2: DANA-FARBER CANCER INSTITUTE PRINCIPLES OF A FAIR, NONPUNITIVE, AND JUST CULTURE
Background

It is inevitable that people will make mistakes or experience misunderstandings in any work environment. When events occur that cause harm, or have the potential to cause harm to patients or staff members, or that place the Institute at legal, financial or ethical risk, a choice exists: to learn or to blame. Dana-Farber Cancer Institute is committed to creating a work environment that emphasizes learning rather than blame.

Dana-Farber Cancer Institute recognizes the complexity and interdependence of the work environment in all aspects of its operations, including patient care, clinical operations, research, support services and administration. The intent is to promote an atmosphere where any employee can openly discuss errors of commission or omission, process improvements, and/or systems corrections without the fear of reprisal.

It is well documented that most errors, whether or not they cause harm, are due to breakdowns in organizational systems; however, when an error takes place, individual culprits are often sought. Blaming individuals creates a culture of fear and defensiveness that diminishes both learning and the capacity to constantly improve systems.

Most errors take place within systems that themselves contribute to the error. In spite of this, it is difficult to create an institutional culture that integrates the understanding that systems failures are the root cause of most errors. Learning from errors often points to beneficial changes in systems and management processes as well as in individual behavior.

In the context of promoting a fair and just culture, what does it mean? A fair and just culture means giving constructive feedback and critical analysis in skillful ways, doing assessments that are based on facts, and having respect for the complexity of the situation. It also means providing fair-minded treatment, having productive conversations, and creating effective structures that help people reveal their errors and help the organization learn from them. A fair and just culture does *not* mean non-accountable, nor does it mean an avoidance of critique or assessment of competence. Rather, when incompetence or substandard performance is revealed after careful collection of facts, and/or there is reckless or willful violation of policies or negligent behavior, corrective or disciplinary action may be appropriate.

Applying these principles creates an opportunity to enact the core values of the Dana-Farber Cancer Institute. In order to have the greatest impact and achieve the highest level of excellence, staff must be able to speak up about problems, errors, conflicts and misunderstandings in an environment where it is the shared goal to identify and discuss problems with curiosity and respect. To achieve excellence, unwanted or unexpected outcomes and inefficiencies of practice must be used as the basis for a learning process. Respect must be shown to all people at every level of the organization.

1. DFCI strives to create a learning environment and a workplace that support the core values of impact, excellence, respect/compassion and discovery in every aspect of work at the Institute.
2. DFCI supports the efforts of every individual to deliver the best work possible. When errors are made and/or misunderstandings occur, the Institute strives to establish accountability in the context of the system in which they occurred.

We commit to creating an institutional work environment that is least likely to cause or support error.

We are proactive about identifying system flaws.

3. DFCI commits to holding individuals accountable for their own performance in accordance with their job responsibilities and the DFCI core values. However, individuals should not carry the burden for system flaws over which they had no control.

4. DFCI promotes open interdisciplinary discussion of untoward events (errors, mistakes, misunderstandings or system failures resulting in harm, potential harm or adverse outcome) by all who work, visit or are cared for at the Institute.

We commit to developing and maintaining easily available and simple processes to discuss untoward events.

We commit to eliciting different points of view to identify sources of untoward events and to use the information to improve the working and care environment.

We commit to fostering an interdisciplinary teamwork approach to the analysis of untoward events and to the actions taken to address them.

We believe that individuals are responsible for surfacing untoward events and for contributing to the elimination of system flaws.

We commit to analyzing episodes of institutional or patient harm or potential harm in an unbiased fashion to best determine the contributions of system and individual factors.

We seek solutions that promote simplification and standardization wherever possible.

5. DFCI acts to improve all areas of the workplace by implementing changes based on our analysis of problems and potential or actual harm.

We know that actions designed to address the root causes of untoward events will improve the effectiveness of our work environment and the safety of care. We commit to identifying and assigning responsibility for implementing those actions to specific individuals or groups.

We commit to developing timely and effective follow-up and an effective organizational culture through education and systems for ensuring on-going competency.

6. DFCI commits to a culture of inclusion and education.

We commit to fostering a culture that is concerned with safety in research, clinical care and administration through continuous education, proactive interventions and safety-based leadership.

We believe that patient input is indispensable to the delivery of safe care and we commit to promoting patient and family participation.

7. DFCI will assess our success in promoting a learning environment by evaluating our willingness to communicate openly and by the improvements we achieve.

We commit to monitoring actions and attitudes for their effectiveness in supporting a culture of safety and modifying actions as needed.

[Principles adapted from Allan Frankel, M.D., and the Patient Safety Leaders at Partners Healthcare System]

REFERENCES

1. Wolf GA, Greenhouse PK. Blueprint for design: creating models that direct change. J Nurs Adm 2007;37(9):381–7.

2. Institute of Medicine. Crossing the quality chasm: a new system for the 21st century. Washington, DC: National Academy Press; 2001.

3. Agency for Healthcare Research and Quality and National Institute of Mental Health. Program announcement. Patient centered care: customizing care to meet patients' needs. 2001, July 31. Available at: http://grants.nih.gov/grants/guide/pafiles/PA-01-124.html. Accessed May 15, 2008.

4. Agency for Healthcare Research and Quality. National healthcare quality report, 2006. Available at: http://www.ahrq.gov/qual/hrqr06/nhqr06.htm. Accessed May 15, 2008.

5. Joint Commission. The Joint Commission Hospital Accreditation Program—2009 chapter: national patient safety goals. Available at: http://www.jointcommission.org/NR/rdonlyres/31666E86-E7F4-423E-9BE8-F05BD1CB0AA8/0/09_NPSG_HAP.pdf. Accessed June 18, 2008.

6. Balint M. The doctor, his patient and the illness. London: Pitman Medical; 1964.

7. Gerteis M, Edgman-Levitan S, Daley J, et al. Through the patient's eyes: understanding and promoting patient-centered care. San Francisco (CA): Jossey-Bass Publishers; 1993.

8. Pew-Fetzer Task Force on Advancing Psychosocial Health Education. Tresolini, CP. Health professions, education and relationship-centered care. San

Francisco (CA): Pew Health Professions Commission; 1994.

9. Roter D. The enduring and evolving nature of the patient-physician relationship. Patient Educ Couns 2000;39:5–15.

10. Mead N, Bower P. Patient centeredness: a conceptual framework and review of the empirical literature. Soc Sci Med 2000;51:1087–110.

11. Conway J, Johnson B, Edgman-Levitan S, et al. Partnering with patients and families to design a patient- and family-centered health care system: a roadmap for the future. A work in progress. June 2006. Available at: http://www.familycenteredcare.org/pdf/Roadmap.pdf. Accessed June 25, 2008.

12. Balint E. The possibilities of patient centered medicine. J R Coll Gen Pract 1969;17(82):269–76.

13. Byrne P, Long B. Doctors talking to patients. London: HMSO; 1976.

14. McWhinney I. The need for a transformed clinical method. In: Stewart M, Roter D, editors. Communicating with medical patients. London: Sage; 1989.

15. NRC/Picker. Our philosophy–eight dimensions. Available at: http://www.nrcpicker.com/Measurement/Understanding%20PCC/Pages/default.aspx. Accessed June 18, 2008.

16. Winefield H, Murrell T, Clifford J, et al. The search for reliable and valid measures of patient-centeredness. Psychology and Health 1996;11:811–24.

17. Laine C, Davidoff F. Patient centered medicine: a professional evolution. JAMA 1996;257:152–6.

18. Institute for Family Centered Care. FAQ. Available at: www.familycenteredcare.og/faq.html. Accessed June 18, 2008.

19. Johnson B, Abraham M, Conway J, et al. Partnering with patients and families to design a patient- and family-centered health care system. Cambridge (MA): Institute for Healthcare Improvement; April 2008.

20. Reid Ponte P, Conlin G, Conway JB, et al. Making patient-centered care come alive. J Nurs Adm 2003;3(2):82–90.

21. Titone J, Cross R, Sileo M, et al. Taking family-centered care to a higher level on the heart and kidney unit. Pediatr Nurs 2004;30:495–7.

22. Hobbs SF, Sodomka PF. Developing partnerships among patients, families, and staff at the Medical College of Georgia Hospital and Clinics. Jt Comm J Qual Improv 2000;26:268–76.

23. Smith T, Conant Rees HL. Making family-centered care a reality. Semin Nurs Manag 2000;8(3):136–42.

24. Stewart M, Brown JB, Donner A, et al. Impact of patient centered care on outcomes. J Fam Pract 2000;49:796–804.

25. van Ryn M, Fu SS. Paved with good intentions: do public health and human service providers contribute to racial/ethnic disparities in health? Am J Public Health 2003;93(2):248–55.

26. Institute of Medicine. To err is human: building a safer health system. Washington, DC: National Academies Press; 2000.

27. Agency for Healthcare Research and Quality. Making health care safer: a critical analysis of patient safety practices. Evidence report/technology assessment: number 43. AHRQ publication no. 01–E058. July 2001. Available at: http://www.ahrq.gov/clinic/patsafety/. Accessed May 15, 2008.

28. Schuster MA, McGlynn EA, Brook RH. How good is the quality of health care in the United States? Milbank Q 1998;76(4):517–63.

29. Schuster MA, McGlynn EA, Brook RH. How good is the quality of health care in the United States? Milbank Q 2005;83(4):843–95.

30. Herzog A, Hart C. A culture of safety: how to achieve it. Psychiatry online.org Available at: http://pn.psychiatryonline.org/cgi/content/full/39/4/81. Accessed June 18, 2008.

31. Kizer K. Extreme makeover: the case of VA healthcare. Presented at Intermountain Health Care Advanced Training Program in Quality and Safety. April 30, 2008; Salt Lake City, Utah.

32. Reid Ponte P, Connor M, DeMarco R, et al. Linking patient- and family-centered care and patient safety: the next leap. Nurs Econ 2004;22(4):211–5.

33. Connor M, Ponte PR, Conway J. Multidisciplinary approaches to reducing error and risk in a patient care setting. Crit Care Nurs Clin North Am 2002; 14(4):359–67, viii.

34. Conway J, Nathan D, Benz E, et al. Key learning from the Dana-Farber Cancer Institute's 10-year patient safety journey. American Society of Clinical Oncology 2006 educational book. Alexandria (VA): American Society of Clinical Oncology; 2006.

35. Reid Ponte P. Nurse-physician co-leadership: a model of interdisciplinary practice governance. J Nurs Adm 2004;34(11):481–4.

36. Reid Ponte P. Personal. In: Adams Thompson L, O'Neil EH, editors. The nurse executive: the four principles of management. NY: Springer Publishing Company; 2008. p. 217–41.

37. Connor M, Duncombe D, Barclay E, et al. Creating a fair and just culture: one institution's path toward organizational change. Jt Comm J Qual Patient Saf 2007;33(10):617–24.

38. Gittell JH. Cost/quality tradeoffs in the departure process? evidence from the major U.S. airlines. Transportation Research Record 1995;1480:25–36.

39. Gittell JH. The Southwest Airlines way: using the power of relationships to achieve high performance. New York: McGraw-Hill; 2003.

40. Wolf G, Triolo P, Reid Ponte P. Magnet recognition program: the next generation. J Nurs Adm 2008;38:200–4.

41. McClure M, Poulin M, Sovies M, et al. Magnet hospitals: attraction and retention of professional nurses. Kansas City (MO): American Academy of Nursing; 1983.

42. Scott JG, Sochalski J, Aiken L. Review of magnet hospital research: findings and implications for professional nursing practice. J Nurs Adm 1999;29(1): 9–19.

43. Aiken LH, Gwyther ME, Friese CR. The registered nurse workforce: infrastructure for health reform. Stat Bull Metrop Insur Co 1995;71:2–9.

44. Friese CR. Nurse practice environments and outcomes: implications for oncology nursing. Oncol Nurs Forum 2005;32:765–72.

45. Lake ET, Friese CR. Variations in nursing practice environments: relation to staffing and hospital characteristics. Nurs Res 2006;55:1–9.

46. Friese CR, Lake ET, Aiken LH, et al. Hospital nurse practice environments and outcomes for surgical oncology patients. Health Serv Res 2008;43(4): 1145–63.

47. National Comprehensive Cancer Network. About NCCN. Available at: http://www.nccn.org/about/default.asp. Accessed June 18, 2008.

Nurturing Innovation in the Critical Care Environment: Transforming Care at the Bedside

Lisa Donahue, DrNP, RN[a],*, Sandra Rader, RN, MSA[a],
Pamela Klauer Triolo, PhD, RN, FAAN[b]

KEYWORDS

- Innovation • Transforming care at the bedside
- Patient safety • Staff satisfaction • Efficiency • Critical care

The call to action for creating a safer patient environment was brought to the forefront with the Institute of Medicine (IOM) reports: *To Err is Human*,[1] *Crossing the Quality Chasm*,[2] and *Keeping Patients Safe*.[3] These reports served as the springboard for the public and health care organizations to recognize the flaws present in processes and work environments. This work also served as a catalyst for the efforts of the Robert Wood Johnson Foundation (RWJF) and the Institute of Healthcare Improvement (IHI) to join forces in the creation of the Transforming Care at the Bedside (TCAB) project. The purpose of the TCAB project was to recognize the value of front-line staff and their contribution toward ensuring the quality of hospital care.[4] Although the focus began on medical-surgical units, those involved with the work recognized the value of this innovative improvement strategy across the hospital, including critical care units. Most recently, the TCAB project transitioned from RWJF and IHI sponsorship to the American Organization of Nurse Executives (AONE). The purpose of this article is to discuss implementation of the TCAB project at UPMC Shadyside as the vehicle to nurture care delivery innovation across settings in acute and critical care.

OVERVIEW

UPMC Shadyside is a 517–licensed-bed tertiary care hospital located in Pittsburgh. It serves as one of the flagship hospitals. UPMC is a fully integrated health care delivery system of 21 hospitals located in western Pennsylvania and abroad, including hospitals in Palermo, Sicily, and Dublin, Ireland, and it provides the full continuum of care from home care to senior living. UPMC employs more than 48,000 staff, of whom 11,000 are nurses. UPMC also includes a health plan and three diploma schools of nursing, one of which is the Shadyside School of Nursing.

The organizational culture at UPMC Shadyside has traditionally embraced and valued change. Shadyside's focus in disruptive innovation began in 1998 with the first clinical design initiative. A few years later, the hospital created a care team to redesign processes using the Toyota model. This work immediately followed the IOM's call to action in 2001 to improve health care.[2] Therefore, the opportunity to serve as one of the original TCAB project sites across the country was a natural fit for UPMC Shadyside.

The goal of the collaboration with the RWJF and IHI was to generate and test changes to improve

a Patient Care Services, UPMC Shadyside, 5230 Centre Avenue, Pittsburgh, PA 15232, USA
b UPMC, 11037 Forbes Tower, 200 Lothrop Street, Pittsburgh, PA 15213, USA
* Corresponding author.
E-mail address: donahuela2@upmc.edu (L. Donahue).

Crit Care Nurs Clin N Am 20 (2008) 465–469
doi:10.1016/j.ccell.2008.08.009

care delivery on Medical-Surgical units while also improving staff satisfaction.[5] The TCAB project took shape in 2003. UPMC Shadyside joined two other hospitals, Kaiser Permanente (Roseville, California) and Seton Northwest Hospital (Austin, Texas), to begin the TCAB journey under the direction of the RWJF and IHI. The journey worked to engage front-line staff in problem identification through a brain-storming process called a "deep dive."[5] The deep dive then opened the doors toward creating solutions at the point of care. What followed were rapid tests of change around the ideas generated. Issues and improvements were based on the dimensions of quality as defined by the IOM and then translated as the tenents of the TCAB project: safe and reliable care, vitality and teamwork, patient-centered care, and value-added care processes.[5]

The TCAB project identifies safe and reliable care as known and tested best practices. Staff vitality has been recognized as an environment that promotes staff support while nurturing professional growth and development, and striving for excellence in health care. The aim of patient centeredness is the care of the whole person and family with respect to individual values while maintaining continuity of care. Finally, value-added processes aim to reduce waste through the redesign of work, care provision processes, or physical space to promote a continuous flow of patient care.[6]

TCAB promotes the patient and family experience in addition to the experience of their health care providers.[4] UPMC Shadyside depicts this agenda as creating the hospital of the future, wherein the right care is provided to the right patient at the right time in the right way every time.

The TCAB project infrastructure for continuous innovation was supported by the creation of improvement specialists and "champions of change" supporting all departments. The improvement specialists serve as the support personnel and resident TCAB experts. The champions of change are a group of unit-based representatives who have completed a brief education program in the TCAB principles labeled "TCAB 101." The improvement specialists are available in a consultative role to the unit-based staff directly engaged in the work. They assist through observations, collection of compliance and related safety data, and outcome reporting, all this while spearheading process improvements along the way. An example of their work has been the development and rollout of a safe patient hand-off initiative called "Ticket to Ride." The improvement specialists facilitated the creation of a hand-off report form used by departments as patients move from department to department. Another example of their work has been around the medication reconciliation process. They work with nurses and physicians to identify necessary automated and manual process improvements.

The heart of the work rests with the champions of change. It is through them that the TCAB project lives and breathes on individual nursing units. They are the unit-based front-line staff members who serve as the liaison between staff and the improvement specialists. They assist in generating tests of change on their units with staff involvement to address issues identified on the unit-based "deep dive."

Because the TCAB project began as an initiative to redesign care, one of the first and most successful TCAB initiatives brought rapid response teams to the bedside during medical crises.[7] UPMC Shadyside took that a step further in their development of Condition H (Help), allowing patients and families the opportunity to summon a rapid response team. Condition H is a patient safety program developed at UPMC Shadyside through the collaboration of Tami Merryman, Vice-President of the UPMC Center for Quality Improvement and Innovation, and Sorrel King. As the mother of an 18-month-old daughter, Sorrel recognized the need for a patient/family-initiated rapid response team. Her daughter, Josie, lost her life because of a series of events and multiple breakdowns in communication in a health care facility. Born of this tragic event, Condition H enables patients or family members to activate a rapid response team if they believe there is an emergency or a noticeable clinical change or if they have serious concerns regarding how care is being given, managed, or planned. Condition H asks patients and visitors to be part of the care team by alerting caregivers to clinical changes.[8]

Nurses educate patients about the Condition H program on admission. Every Condition H call brings a rapid response team immediately to the patient's bedside. The response team at UPMC Shadyside consists of a house physician (internal medicine), the administrative nursing coordinator, and a patient relations coordinator (PRC). The PRC conducts a follow-up interview with the patient or family 24 hours after the call to determine the patient's perception of the quality of the response and ensure that the resolution has remained effective. In nearly all cases, the patient or family has expressed satisfaction with the response to the call and with the actions taken to remedy the concerns. UPMC Shadyside has guided or assisted each of the other UPMC business units in setting up and launching similar

Condition H programs. This program at UPMC Shadyside has served as a model and resource for hospitals across the country.

ENCULTURATION

The successful integration of the TCAB project on 4-East (the original TCAB unit) set staff members on the inevitable course to spread TCAB to the additional 13 medical-surgical units of the hospital. This expansion was not only successful but promoted a heightened sense of meaning, purpose, direction, and innovation for all the nursing units. Born of the enthusiastic embrace of the TCAB project was incredible work driven by the nurses at the bedside. This work included such initiatives as pain management posters, patient medication schedules for home use, and staff vitality huddles. Because the nursing work flow uses computerized medication carts and geographic patient care assignments, the staff of one medical-surgical unit identified the loss of collegiality. To remedy this situation, they developed the concept of the staff vitality huddle. Huddles occur between 9:30 and 10:00 AM, calling all nurses to the workroom near the nurses' station. They spend 10 to 15 minutes to network while nothing clinical is discussed. Five to eight nurses attend each time, and huddles occur three to five times per week. It has had an overwhelmingly positive effect on the staff. Huddles have now spread to the evening shift. One hundred percent of the nurses surveyed stated the huddles should continue.

The TCAB project units continued to incorporate TCAB philosophies into their daily practice and recognize the value of TCAB as the vehicle to elicit change and promote improved outcomes. The development of the TCAB champions, the commitment from the unit directors, and the involvement of the staff provided the supportive infrastructure necessary to take the next step: the invitation for the five intensive care units (ICUs) to join the TCAB project journey. They accepted.

NEXT GENERATION OF TRANSFORMING CARE AT THE BEDSIDE

Generally, intensive care nurses are viewed as critical thinkers with the flexibility to adapt and decisively manage critical situations. These qualities contribute to their successes in caring for those critically ill patients in that ever-changing environment. Critical care nurses possess the ability to speak up, initiate changes when issues are recognized, and advocate for a position they believe in. They also acclimate swiftly, make intuitive decisions, and think on their feet. These qualities

create a natural environment to cultivate TCAB as the vehicle for process improvement.

The first barrier of the TCAB project spread to critical care was the perception that this was asking for additional work. The challenge was to demonstrate to the ICU nurses that TCAB was simply a vehicle to package much of the work that they were already doing into a logical and quality-focused product with proven results. Also key to successful enculturation was the understanding of the TCAB project applications in the areas of process improvement to promote safe and reliable care, staff vitality, patient-centered care, and value-added processes free of waste.

The Surgical-Oncology ICU (SICU) was led down the TCAB project path in the year before the spread. The new unit director was familiar with the TCAB project and was interested in the application of those principles on her unit. She introduced the concepts early and began promoting small successful tests of change. Having been a staff nurse in that unit and now a unit leader, she was required to change her role from that of a participant to that of an observer. She truly defined the "art of observation" by recognizing many of their issues with the hunting and gathering of equipment and supplies. Her ability to step back, watch, and encourage the staff to develop a plan for improvement was in the true spirit of TCAB. The staff identified a problem, dug deep to identify the "why's" of the situation, developed and implemented a plan, and evaluated the results. This team was ready to take the ball and run, and since the spread of TCAB to the ICUs, they have done just that. The staff implemented many successful strategies with supply placement on the unit to decrease hunting and gathering. They have also solved their issue of lost laboratory labels through the use of a tackle box labeled with the patient room numbers. This is just one more example of simple straightforward tests of change that can dramatically affect the flow of patient care and unnecessary work by the staff.

It was evident that a crucial component to the successful spread of TCAB to the ICU units was to provide examples of how they functioned as "TCABers" already. As far back as 2006, the Medical-Surgical ICU (MSICU) had an understanding of patient-centered initiatives to improve patient outcomes and patient and staff satisfaction. In the true spirit of the TCAB philosophies, the staff worked to develop a program called the Clinical Partnership Program (CPP). This is a collaborative effort between the ICU and the step-down areas that receive the ICU's patients once they are able to be transferred from the ICU environment. The patients are identified based on acuity and complexity. The selected patients, the ICU nurse, the bedside nurse, and resident (when appropriate) have ongoing communication and patient assessment support as long as necessary. Support may be in terms of assistance with complex dressings, physical assessment, and continuation of plan of care. The multifaceted goals of this collaborative effort include (1) to improve patient satisfaction; (2) to decrease adverse outcomes (respiratory failure, acute renal failure, and stroke); (3) to decrease length of stay; (4) to improve nursing satisfaction; (5) to avert readmissions to the ICU; (6) to improve collegial relationships between MSICU and Medical-Surgical nurses; (7) to promote continuity of care; (8) to decrease patient mortality; and (9) to decrease the number of crisis events, such as Condition C's and A's. Crisis events are defined as a Condition C when a crisis event requires intervention (eg, respiratory or other emergent events). Condition "C" should be called whenever an unstable patient needs rapid evaluation and treatment. This includes any potentially life-threatening condition other than cardiopulmonary arrest and is not limited to acute respiratory distress or hemodynamic instability. In the event that the patient needs to be transferred to a monitored bed or ICU, the Condition C team is responsible for transporting the patient. The crucial aspect of a Condition C is early request for assistance. Condition A is defined as an event that requires cardiopulmonary resuscitation (CPR).[9]

The appropriate placement of a patient in the CPP is determined by the ICU nurse caring for the patient. An order for the clinical partnership is placed on the patient record. Documentation occurs in the Interdisciplinary Plan of Care (IPOC) section of the chart as a "Complicated Patient Recovery" issue and a "Collaborative Practice" goal with the medical-surgical ICU. Once transferred from the ICU, the patient is seen each day by a nurse from the ICU and through discussion and collaboration with the medical-surgical unit nurse, the patient plan of care is determined. Those daily visits are then documented in the IPOC and include assessment, patient progress, emotional well-being, family interaction, and other pertinent patient information. A patient is followed on the CCP until it is determined that it is no longer necessary or the patient is close to discharge.

As of December 2007, the review of outcomes was outstanding. By that date, there were 103 patients who participated in the CPP with no Condition C's or A's. Only 2 patients returned to the ICU. These patients were identified early and returned to ICU before deterioration to a Condition C. Of those patients returned to the ICU, nurses familiar

with them followed them throughout their continuum of care. This level of continuity promoted a feeling of safety and security for the patients and their families and contributed to staff satisfaction. The CPP initiative has since spread to all the ICU units. Each critical care unit and its partner medical-surgical unit have adopted this program to meet the needs of their patients, families, and staff.

Innovations from the TCAB project range from the complex to the obviously simple but important. The Neuroscience ICU (NSICU) staff has also identified areas for process improvement in the waste associated with stocking isolation rooms. The staff determined that placing their patient care supplies in roving carts outside the patient doorway would serve two purposes. Primarily, it decreased the amount of waste created when an isolation patient was moved and the supplies were discarded. It also provided the nurses with many necessary supplies close at hand that were normally in a central location. This new process was implemented even before the spread of the TCAB project to the ICUs. During the "TCAB 101" educational sessions held throughout the initial rollout, the identifiers of metrics were explained and the TCAB project unfolded. The NSICU nurses already recognized the waste (value-added processes) and the need for mobility of care supplies (staff vitality). The staff desire to stop the waste of unused supplies and decrease hunting and gathering for those supplies was the driving force for this work flow redesign. The metrics of this change were defined by sheer accident. In just monitoring stock use, it has been evident that there is less waste. At this writing, the financial analysis to demonstrate the cost savings accurately is being calculated. The correlation of this project to the TCAB project process provided the business case in addition to staff satisfaction to support the initiative. Once staff were able to understand the process and apply it to work they had already done, enlightenment followed.

The Cardiothoracic ICU (CTICU) embarked on an even larger project. With the support and assistance from the director of enterostomal therapy and an advanced practice nurse, they implemented a case study analysis on the skin care breakdown of patients who underwent open-heart surgery. The prevention of skin breakdown in this patient population was a challenge recognized by the front-line staff. Lengthy operating times in conjunction with immobility and decreased perfusion are known contributing factors to compromised skin integrity.[10] It has been well documented that this compromise leads to longer hospital stays, poor patient outcomes, and a negative perception of care.[10]

The staff identified ways to combat skin care breakdown and initiated a pilot study to keep the patient who underwent open-heart surgery off of his or her back for the first 12 hours after surgery. Although a challenge in many patients because of hemodynamic instability, the guidelines for safe practice were established and the pilot project was moved forward. In the CTICU, applying the TCAB principles to the work staff members were already doing was equally enlightening. The staff had already appreciated the metrics (increased length of stay and poor patient outcomes) and developed a plan to test in the hope of improving those outcomes (patient-centered care). Anecdotal findings suggested that active participation in work redesign promoted an improved level of pride and satisfaction in their work (staff vitality).[6]

The CTICU staff had already fully expressed a TCAB project test of change before even thoroughly understanding the dynamics of the process. As an example, the application of TCAB principles to a project they had already completed was a winning situation and eye-opening experience. The compilation of the data from a pilot study of this magnitude requires meticulous review of the patient's condition and nursing documentation. As staff anxiously anticipated the tally of those results, one thing became clear. The increased awareness regarding skin care issues in conjunction with the enhanced surveillance were the driving forces towards improved outcomes. The unit has since participated in the decision-making process for new mattresses and is integrally involved in skin care product evaluations.

SUMMARY

Critical care nurses, because of their penchant for action and risk taking, are naturals for process improvement. The recognition of their valued opinions and ideas, along with absorption of the TCAB philosophies, has been the foundation for the successful spread of the TCAB initiative to the ICUs at UPMC Shadyside. Although in the early phases of

implementation, the enthusiasm toward participation and growth is evident. The resulting momentum toward ongoing process improvement supports the promise of a bright future for the TCAB project in the world of critical care.

REFERENCES

1. Committee on Quality of Health Care in America. In: Kohn LT, Corrigan JM, Donaldson MS, editors. To err is human: building a safety health system. Washington, DC: National Academics Press; 2000.
2. Committee on Quality of Health Care in America and Institute of Medicine. Crossing the quality chasm: a new health system in the 21st century. Washington, DC: National Academics Press; 2001.
3. Committee on Quality of Health Care in America and Institute of Medicine. Keeping patients safe: transforming the work environment of nurses. Washington, DC: National Academics Press; 2003.
4. Rutherford P, Lee B, Greiner A. Transforming care at the bedside. IHI innovation series white paper. Boston: Institute for Healthcare Improvement; 2004.
5. Viney M, Batcheller J, Houston S, et al. Transforming care at the bedside: designing new care systems in an age of complexity. J Nurs Care Qual 2006;21(2):143–50.
6. Transforming care at the bedside: using a team approach to give nurses—and their patients—new voices in providing high-quality care. Qual Lett Healthc Lead 2005;17(11):2–8.
7. Scholle C, Mininni N. How rapid response teams save lives. Nursing 2006;36(1):36–40.
8. Greenhouse PK, Kuzminsky B, Martin SC, et al. Calling a condition H(elp). Am J Nurs 2006;106(11):63–6.
9. University of Pittsburgh Medical Center. (2002) Resuscitation (Condition A) and medical crisis management (Condition C) (policy). Available at: http://policymanuals.infonet.upmc.com/PresbyShadyNursing. Accessed June 1, 2008.
10. Courtney BA, Ruppman JB, Cooper HM. Save our skin: initiative cuts pressure ulcer incidence in half. Nurs Manag 2006;37(4):36–45.

Simulation as a Vehicle for Enhancing Collaborative Practice Models

Pamela R. Jeffries, DNS, RN, FAAN, ANEF[a],*,
Angela M. McNelis, PhD, RN[b], Corinne A. Wheeler, PhD, RN[b]

KEYWORDS

- Clinical simulation • Collaborative practice models
- Educational technology • Interdisciplinary collaboration
- Interdisciplinary learning

Health care professionals need to be prepared for safe and efficient practice and for collaborating effectively with practitioners from other disciplines. Faced with these challenges, educators must explore innovative ways to teach medical, nursing, and other health care students and professionals how to work together to deliver care in real-world clinical practice. Developments in educational technology make a wide array of options available to facilitate this preparation. These developments also create an advantageous environment for systematic and substantial change, including a focus on interdisciplinary, collaborative learning. Lectures and small-group work can impart technical knowledge but are inadequate to prepare students for the complexities of the work place or for working collaboratively. Clinical simulation used in a collaborative practice approach is a powerful tool to prepare health care providers for shared responsibility for patient care.[1]

Clinical simulations in professional curricula are being used increasingly to prepare providers for quality practice, but little is known about how these simulations can be used to foster collaborative practice across disciplines. This article provides an overview of what simulation is, what collaborative practice models are, and how to set up a model using simulations. An example of a collaborative practice model is presented, and nursing implications of using a collaborative practice model in simulations are discussed.

SIMULATION DEFINITION, PURPOSES, AND USES

Simulation, in specific reference to health care, is an attempt to replicate essential aspects of a clinical scenario so that when a similar scenario occurs in a clinical setting, the situation can be managed readily and successfully.[2] The educator decides if the simulation will focus on the process of teaching–learning and progress toward an outcome (formative) or on the attainment of the learning objectives (summative).

When simulations are used in a formative manner, as in a teaching–learning activity, the goal is to improve student performance. In this situation, students receive feedback from the educator and from peers, and they reflect on their knowledge, skills, and critical thinking relative to the simulation. When simulations are used in a collaborative practice approach, students are exposed to the knowledge, skills, and critical thinking of practitioners outside their own discipline and can begin to appreciate the contributions each team member can make in patient care.

[a] Department of Adult Health, Indiana University School of Nursing, Indiana University School of Nursing, 1111 Middle Drive, NU140, Indianapolis, IN 46202, USA
[b] Department of Environments for Health, Indiana University School of Nursing; Indiana University School of Nursing, 1111 Middle Drive, NU403H, Indianapolis, IN 46202, USA
* Corresponding author.
E-mail address: prjeffri@iupui.edu (P.R. Jeffries).

Crit Care Nurs Clin N Am 20 (2008) 471–480
doi:10.1016/j.ccell.2008.08.005

When simulations are used summatively, feedback about the attainment of learning objectives and/or final competency goals is provided at the conclusion of the teaching–learning activity. The summative approach often becomes a component of progression in a course or program. Summative simulations address the charge by the Institute of Medicine[3] to improve patient care by increasing collaboration among clinicians in practice settings. Educational initiatives that encourage teamwork among the health care disciplines are critical to performing this mission.

COLLABORATIVE PRACTICE MODELS
Overview

In today's health care system, no profession or discipline can operate alone. Interdisciplinary collaboration is vital for creating a safe system of care. Health care providers need to understand that teamwork and communication reduce errors.[4] Quality client outcomes rely on professional teamwork, and the level of collaboration that takes place can affect safety outcomes directly.[5]

Studies among professional health science students have shown a strong relationship between communication skills and teamwork training, with such skills leading to fewer errors, improved patient satisfaction, and more timely clinical decision-making in critical client events.[6–8] To promote a "culture of safety," the Institute of Medicine (IOM), the Joint Commission (formerly the Joint Commission on Accreditation of Healthcare Organizations), and others have encouraged health care professionals to improve communication and teamwork.

Traditionally, the education of health care professionals has been from a discipline specific, rather than interdisciplinary approach. Faculty in the health sciences now are adopting an evidence-based model of teaching in an integrated manner that enables students to learn to communicate and make clinical decisions collaboratively.[9] Communication among nurses and physicians and others does not "just happen" in a clinical setting; it is a skill that must be taught during professional education.

Collaborative practice has been defined as an interprofessional process for communication and decision-making that enables the separate and shared knowledge and skills of care providers to influence synergistically the client care provided. Essentials needed for collaborative work include responsibility, accountability, coordination, communication, cooperation, risk-taking, assertiveness, autonomy, and mutual trust and respect.[5,7,10] According to Keleher,[10] the foundational components required to build a successful collaborative practice are a willingness to move beyond basic information-sharing and the ability to challenge distortions and assumptions, using a belief system based on critical self-reflection.

Purposes

Interdisciplinary education is a critical element in improving patient safety.[3] The IOM report identified five essential competencies in this area necessary for health care providers: patient-centered care, interdisciplinary teamwork, evidence-based practice, quality improvement practices, and informatics. Core curricular content that targets patient safety and the use of teaching strategies that facilitate attainment of the five core competencies will prepare future health care providers to improve patient safety in complex health care environments. Unfortunately, educational gaps exist for practitioners in many clinical venues, resulting in an increased frequency of medical errors.[3] Immersing students in a collaborative practice environment where health care professionals learn and practice together would promote safer patient care.

In 2003, the IOM released its recommendations on how health care professional education must bridge the quality gap between the expectations for care and the actual quality of care delivered in health care systems today. To build this bridge, skillful, well-educated, innovative health professionals are needed. To begin this effort, educators need to develop an interdisciplinary educational model as a way of developing a sense of community and collaboration among all health care professionals. Key elements in building such a community are communication, teamwork, trust, and collaboration.[11]

The National Patient Safety Foundation[12] calls for health care professionals to identify and create a core body of knowledge, to identify pathways to apply the knowledge, and to foster communications about patient safety to improve patient outcomes. Meeting these standards will require strategic cooperation among health care organizations, schools of nursing, schools of medicine, and other health care disciplines to develop a model for collaborative educational practice models and to conduct research in this area.

Challenges

Barriers to collaborative practice are many. Role ambiguity and confusion, hierarchical relationships, educational differences, gender issues, and culture are all real barriers to creating collaborative relationships.

Role ambiguity and confusion
Sexton and colleagues[13] report that sufficiently trained critical care health professionals often function well individually but fail to work smoothly as a team. The most difficult tasks encountered by an interdisciplinary team include leadership, communication, and cooperation.[13,14] All three of these tasks are necessary for team members to understand better how members of each discipline function independently within their scope of practice but interdependently in a smoothly operating team. Role ambiguity exists when the goals of one's job or the methods of performing it are unclear. Ambiguity sometimes is characterized by confusion about how work performance is valued or what the limits of one's authority and responsibility are. Certain team members may have unclear expectations of another team member, or they may aware of the expectations but personally find them difficult to accept. Role ambiguity can be reduced by open communication and respect shown for the knowledge and skills brought by each discipline.

Hierarchical relationships
The nurse–physician relationship historically has been one of hierarchy and power, with the physician assuming control. In the past, physicians played a dominant role, and nurses played a more subservient role by deferring all client-related decisions to the physician and communicating in a passive way. Even though advances have been made, economics and educational preparation perpetuate this type of nurse–physician relationship.

Economics contributes to the hierarchy, because physicians usually are the revenue generators in health care systems. Physicians can influence the bottom line of organizations by controlling the number of client admissions or procedures done within that organization; thus physicians have inherent power. Nurses often are considered a "cost" to the organization, because their salaries and benefits are paid directly by the organization.

Educational differences
It has long been recommended that students need role models of collaboration, and faculty members have been encouraged to develop interprofessional training opportunities for socialization to promote interdisciplinary collaboration.[15,16] Health care professionals still are being educated separately, however, and as a result may fail to recognize the important roles played by members of other disciplines. Formal education to help team members understand the scope of their colleagues' practice is essential. Collaboration relies on respect and on trust that each person is doing his or her best. Familiarity with the role, skills, and philosophy of care of each discipline also enhances the collaborative relationship.

Gender issues
Historically, physicians were men, and nurses were women. Today, more women are becoming physicians, and more men are becoming nurses. According to the American Medical Association, men and women are almost equally represented in medicine (2000), although nationally only about 5.4% of registered nurses are men.[17] Multiple studies investigating gender and power found that male physicians maintain a dominant role. A study by Zelek and Phillips[18] found that nurses were less likely to speak up to a male physician, whereas the balance of power was more equal and collaborative when both nurse and physician were women. In a qualitative study by Wear and Keck-McNulty,[19] female nurses reported a higher level of collaboration with female physicians than with male physicians.

Culture
Culture describes a person's way of life, including knowledge, values, beliefs, and behaviors. Culture also includes the way people think about and understand the world and their own lives. A specific culture can be reflected in a nation, region, organization, or in the communication and symbols used by an individual.[20] Contrasting values, beliefs, or understandings held by team members from different cultures can be a barrier to successful collaborative practice.

In some ways, nursing and medicine are rooted in different cultures. The respective philosophies represent different priorities in providing care. Students in nursing and medicine are indoctrinated in these diverging philosophies, values, and beliefs early in their educational preparation, making collaboration potentially difficult. Introducing interdisciplinary, collaborative learning into both nursing and medical curricula decreases this ethos dissonance and promotes a culture of collaboration.

Organizations also have their own cultures. An organization that values teamwork and communication provides an environment supportive of collaboration among disciplines. Other organizations may have a rich tradition of social order that supports a hierarchical system.[5]

Benefits of the collaborative practice model
Research has demonstrated positive outcomes from interdisciplinary collaboration for both health

care providers and patients.[6,21,22] Collaborative practice models are known to improve patient safety, patient satisfaction, care coordination, and health care provider working relationships. They also lead to more efficient use of time, decreased length of hospital stays, and reduced cost.[5,10] Collaborative practice allows the full skill sets of the team to be used and facilitates continued learning for all team members.

SETTING UP A COLLABORATIVE PRACTICE MODEL USING SIMULATIONS
Collaborative Learning with Simulations

Although communication skills may be learned by trial and error in a clinical setting, a formal approach to instruction has been shown to be more efficient and to enhance student confidence.[8] Collaborative learning with simulations also has been found to increase a sense of collegiality and teamwork.[23] One way to develop mutual respect, to enhance communication, and to improve relationships among disciplines is to involve the members of the various disciplines in a group-learning simulation experience.

Simulation Design Overview

The design for creating an interdisciplinary teaching simulation must be appropriate for all the disciplines involved in the activity. Although course

goals and skill competencies may differ among disciplines, the learning outcomes of the simulation (eg, communication skills) may apply to all. Each simulation design, regardless of discipline, should include the following characteristics: objectives, roles, fidelity, problem-solving, support, and guided reflection.[24] The evaluation of each simulation process should include an assessment of each of these design features as well as learning outcomes related to collaborative practice. **Fig. 1** is an example of a collaborative model used at the Indiana University Schools of Nursing and Medicine.

Characteristics of a Simulation Design

Objectives
Before participating in a simulation experience, learners need to be provided with information regarding its purpose and objectives. Pre-simulation information can be sent to students several days before the event to help them prepare for the experience. Objectives for the activity need to be provided clearly to the learner; they must state the intended outcome(s) of the experience, expected learner behaviors, and enough detail to allow the learner to participate in the event effectively.[24] It is best to limit each simulation to no more than two or three main objectives. During the debriefing session following the simulation

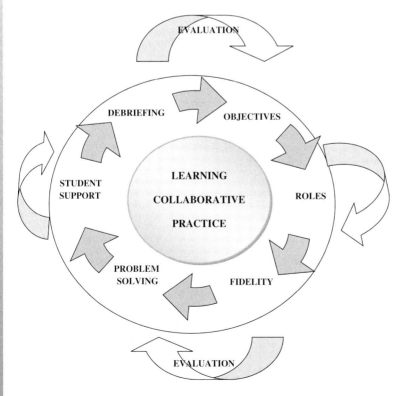

Fig. 1. Characteristics of an interdisciplinary teaching simulation.

event, the objectives can be revisited to explore with the students how they felt the objectives were met.

Roles

Regardless of the fidelity (realism) or complexity of the simulation, the two constant roles are those of educator and student. Depending on the simulation design, other roles may include actors playing the part of a standardized patient or family member and support staff assisting with room set-up for high-fidelity technology.

The specifics of the faculty role are determined by whether the simulation is designed for student learning or evaluation. When the goal is learning, the faculty member is involved more actively in supporting the student by providing information before the simulation or by providing "cues" during the actual simulation activity. If the goal is evaluation, the faculty takes on the role of observer. Whether for learning or evaluations, faculty responsibilities are the same for the design and implementation of the simulation (**Table 1**).

Student roles vary depending on the simulation design. According to Cioffi,[25] clinical student roles are either process-based or response-based. In a process-based role, the student is an active participant and influences the sequence of events (eg, when using a simulator or role-playing in a scenario). The student in a response-based role

does not become actively involved in controlling the event. An example of a response-based role is reviewing a standardized case report and discussing the findings.

In an interdisciplinary simulation, students take on process-based roles. During the simulation activity, a role might be that of the health care provider in one's discipline, or the design might call for a student to take on a role of actor or an observer. Whatever the role assigned, all participants must be prepared for their parts before the activity. It also is expected that each student will be engaged actively throughout the simulation activity and debriefing process.

Fidelity

Human mannequin simulators can perform at three levels of fidelity and sophistication (high, moderate, and low).[26] Fidelity is the extent to which a simulation mimics reality. The high-fidelity mannequin can mimic a real-life situation with interactive features (eg, the mannequin speaks, the chest moves up and down, skin color changes). A moderate-fidelity mannequin may produce audible heart and lung sounds but does not have as high a level of technical sophistication. The low-fidelity mannequin is sometimes referred to as a "static mannequin." It may appear real but has no mechanical features such as voice or lung and heart sounds.[27]

Table 1
Simulation roles and responsibilities

Faculty Role	Student Role			
	Caregiver	Actor	Observer	Other
Provide learner support throughout simulation activity and debriefing	Responsible for own learning	Responsible for own learning	Responsible for own learning	Participate as an actor or observer
Design simulation				
Provide information to the students before the simulation	Engage actively a as health care provider	Engage actively as an actor in designated role	Observe silently, take notes during simulation activity	Provide technology support
Equipment set-up		Give cues		Assist with equipment set-up
Program high-fidelity technology	Self reflection and evaluation	Self reflection and evaluation	Self reflection and evaluation	
Observation				
Evaluate all dimensions of the simulation	Can rotate through assigned roles in addition to talking about the roles during debriefing and reflection.			

In a discussion of teaching teamwork skills in health care, researchers Beaubien and Baker[28] state that high-fidelity simulation is only one of many tools that may be effective. They describe three dimensions of fidelity: environment, equipment, and psychologic, and they propose that psychologic fidelity is the most important for team training. A focus on realism in all aspects of the simulation, not just on the realism of the mannequin, is important.

Health care educators must consider factors beyond providing realistic equipment when designing the collaborative clinical simulations. Learners quickly can become engaged in caring for a human patient mannequin with lung sounds, chest tubes, and real-life heart sounds, but there is more to a successful simulation than the mannequin. What learners are thinking and feeling during the simulation must be considered also. The simulation scenario must call for the use of evidence-based findings, critical thinking, and problem-solving skills related to patient care.

Problem-solving

The design of the simulation ranges from simple to complex and should correspond to the level of problem-solving and decision-making expected of the student. The simulation activity is designed to be aligned with the learner's current knowledge and skill level and to incorporate different levels of uncertainty. The simulation needs to challenge the learner but be attainable. If the level of complexity or problem-solving is too high for the learner, the result will be an unfavorable learning experience. In a complex collaborative practice simulation, the learners have an opportunity to communicate, prioritize assessment findings, initiate care within their scope of practice, and perform team and self-evaluations. For example, in a simulation scenario with the focus on collaborative communication and teamwork involving both medical and nursing students, the simulation provides an opportunity to work with members of the other discipline, to respect each other, and to communicate with each other while focusing on patient-centered care. During the debriefing, the simulation participants can reflect on the experience, self-evaluate, and discuss with the instructor what went right and wrong.

Student support

The educator supports student learning differently during each phase of the simulation. In the pre-simulation phase, faculty members prepare students directly for the simulation experience. During this pre-phase period, students learn the purpose of the simulation, the learning objectives, the process, and what the simulation entails. The student experience during this phase will influence how effective the simulation-based training will be.[29]

During the simulation activity, faculty members support students' learning less directly. Faculty members incorporate a number of cues or hints into the design of the scenario that help the students progress to the next step. The cues should offer enough information for the students to continue without interfering with independent or team problem-solving. Cues can take many forms, such as a telephone call, a laboratory report, or statements from a family member or the voice-programmed human simulator. Most importantly, the cues need to be realistic to the case and prompt the participant toward certain actions. During the final phase of the simulation, the educator supports students through guided reflection, also referred to as "debriefing."

Guided reflection

One of the core elements of the simulation experience is the debriefing session. Immediately after the simulation activity, students and faculty engage in a facilitated discussion. The goal of debriefing is to promote reflective thinking and for learning and discussion to occur in a nonthreatening and organized way.[30] To ensure a successful debriefing process and learning experience, the educator or facilitator must provide a supportive environment in which students feel respected, valued, and free to speak openly. The debriefing process allows students to evaluate and assess the situation using their own self-analysis as well as feedback from others. The debriefing also is a time when elements of a scenario's evolution can be tied to theory, practice, and research.

Principles in Promoting Collaborative Work

The implementation of collaborative practice models is expected by many health care organizations and health care regulatory agencies. The structures, systems, and processes within a collaborative practice model are designed to facilitate communication, cooperation, coordination, and teamwork, with trust and equality being pivotal components. Collaborative practice is not intuitive, however. It involves a philosophy that needs to be learned and practiced by all members of the team. Institutions offering health services education recognize this need and are beginning to integrate collaborative practice models into the educational preparation of nurses, physicians, and other health care providers. Hospitals and organizations are transforming the work culture, especially in critical care areas, by training health professionals in collaborative practice.

EXAMPLE OF A CURRENT COLLABORATIVE PRACTICE MODEL

The demands on health care professionals have become more complex because of advances in technology and increased patient acuity in the clinical agencies. Health care providers face increasingly complex patient-care situations; often decisions must be made rapidly in an atmosphere of conflicting or incomplete information. Given this situation, the need for members of the health care team to collaborate effectively is imperative.[31] Such realities challenge nurse educators to develop teaching –learning activities that focus on collaborative care. One strategy suggested by health care educators for developing collaborative practice competencies is the scenario-based simulation.[32] An example of how such simulations have been used to teach interdisciplinary teams using a collaborative practice model is the American Heart Association's model of teaching advanced cardiac life support (ACLS).

ACLS was developed in 1974 as a course to address the need to integrate knowledge and skills in cardiac resuscitation. The ACLS course is one of the oldest multidisciplinary medical training programs in the United States. The course traditionally is taught in 1 or 2 days, the equivalent of 8 to 16 instructional hours Enrollment in the course includes different health professionals including nurses, physicians, respiratory therapists, and others. Since the course began, the advent of the International Guidelines on Cardiopulmonary Resuscitation (CPR) and Emergency Cardiac Care Conference in 2000 resulted in international guidelines for resuscitation. The new guidelines incorporate evidence-based practice using collaborative teams to learn and perform ACLS. With these new guidelines developed for CPR and ACLS courses, a difference in survival rates after CPR has been demonstrated.[33–35]

For ACLS training, teamwork and collaborative practice are incorporated throughout the course. For example, different health care participants work together to learn to perform a successful code, in which a patient has a cardiac arrest or dysrhythmia resulting in a life-or-death situation. Moretti and colleagues[36] reported a study focusing on patients who had a return of spontaneous circulation after resuscitation by ACLS-trained health care providers. The more ACLS-trained members there were participating in the team, the higher was the likelihood of a return of spontaneous circulation in the patients studied.

In addition, the researchers found that with increased numbers of ACLS-trained rescue squads, survival to hospital discharge increased from 20.6% to 31.7%, and long-term survival increased from 0% to 21.9% 1 year after discharge. The results in this research emphasize the importance of health care professionals learning ACLS and also how the collaborative team effort affects in-hospital and long-term survival rates.

In another study by Gilligan and colleagues[37] the researchers found that ACLS-trained nurses performed as well as ACLS-trained emergency senior house officers in a scenario-based simulation of a cardiac arrest. The researchers recommended that if a physician were not present, the ACLS-trained nurse should act as a team leader. According to the researchers, empowering experienced nurses who have had ACLS training to take over and lead the team until the physician arrives and then work as part of a collaborative team actually can increase survival rates, because in most cases the team begins compressions and defibrillation before the physician arrives. This finding emphasizes the need for collaborative practice that has been started in the learning environment where ACLS is being taught. This example serves as a model of collaborative practice in which interdisciplinary groups work together to improve outcomes and patient survival rates.

NURSING IMPLICATIONS OF USING A COLLABORATIVE PRACTICE MODEL IN SIMULATIONS

Physicians, nurses, and other health care professionals must be prepared to create and establish safer and more efficient practice environments. Faced with many challenges today in health care education, educators must explore innovative ways to teach medical, nursing, and other health care professional students the skills they will need in real-world clinical practice in a cost-effective, productive, and high-quality manner. Discoveries and developments in educational technology make a wide array of options available to faculty to facilitate experiential learning (eg, using sophisticated simulators). Such developments also create an environment ripe for systematic and substantial change. Providing students with limited clinical experiences and immersing them in lecture content and small-group work may impart the requisite technical knowledge; however, this mode of instruction is inadequate to prepare students for the complexities of the work place. Clinical simulation based on a collaborative practice model, as discussed, clinical experience, and experiential teaching methods are powerful tools to prepare competent health care professionals for clinical practice.[1] Health care providers such as hospitals have noted gaps in communication and teamwork. Teamwork solutions are available, but educators must be prepared to develop and implement solutions using a collaborative model.

Teaching strategies and opportunities for implementing collaborative practice models in education are shown in **Table 2**. In accordance with the IOM 2003 recommendations,[3] collaborative practice should be incorporated into the educational arena before students graduate and begin to practice in a real-world environment where collaborative working relationships are imperative. Educators of health care professionals should consider incorporating interdisciplinary simulations into the laboratory and/or clinical practicum experiences. Content and interdisciplinary experiences can be included in student clinical experiences, orientations, and staff development at health care institutions both to promote a culture

of patient safety and interdisciplinary collaboration and also to improve other patient outcomes. Faculty development also must be considered when integrating models of collaborative practice. Faculty members need knowledge and skills to create experiences that include working in partnership with other disciplines, instructors, and students in health care professions. Four key faculty development elements that need to be considered when using simulations are

1. Developing knowledge in designing, developing, and implementing interdisciplinary simulations
2. Establishing guidelines and procedures on how the collaboration will work, taking into account all stakeholders involved (eg, equal partners in decision-making, scheduling laboratory time, sharing resources)
3. Developing a conceptual collaborative model with goals and direction (see **Fig. 1**)

Table 2
Teaching strategies to implement a collaborative practice model

Teaching Strategy	Concept	Potential Outcome Measures
Develop an interdisciplinary simulation to focus on communication skills and collaborative teamwork.	Interdisciplinary communication and collaboration	Collaboration Scale Communication Scale (IUSM, 2008)[27]
Develop an interdisciplinary course in which medical students and nursing students are enrolled to study common concepts and content.	Example of health care ethics, studying the principles of ethics and discussing ethical dilemmas and issues	Focus groups, pre/post testing; develop a simulation dealing with an ethical dilemma and review for selected competencies desired
Set up lunch times, evening events, or other selected times when multidisciplinary students can mix, discuss different concepts, and develop a respect for each discipline and individual.	Mutual respect for each other and the discipline; learn more about the other discipline and the knowledge and skill sets of other team members	Respect instrument measuring respect for other disciplines; conduct focus groups and review reflective journals for concepts desired
Incorporate Web-based discussion forums in which a collaborative team of professionals respond to a specific issue or scenario	Collaborative practice using an online platform to discuss and consider interdisciplinary practice and patient care	Online learning as a platform for teaching interdisciplinary concepts and collaborative practice
Develop and implement Web-based modules on content that are similar for all health care professionals (eg, patient safety) and have the students complete the modules before simulations or other clinical practice	Concepts included in the Web-based module could vary according to the needs of the course, the program competencies, and other variables, but ideas could include patient safety, communication, and health care ethics	Online learning and module competencies defined within the Web-based module could evaluate the concepts via an interdisciplinary simulation designed to assess the concept taught, (eg, culture of safety, authority gradient)

4. Establishing dates and meeting times for the collaborative work, goals, and activities to be discussed and reflected upon

Current college students, sometimes referred to as the "net generation" or "millennials" are more hands-on and active learners, multitaskers, and collaborators who embrace technology as a way of learning and communicating. Millennials like to work in teams with peer-to-peer collaboration.[38] As faculty members learn more about developing simulations and building experiences around a collaborative practice model, it is important to understand learners' characteristics so that educational needs, learning styles, and teaching modalities are considered. With the need for collaborative practice models and the desire to promote better patient outcomes and safer patient care environments, faculty development related to simulation pedagogy is important. To promote collaborative practice, educators must be encouraged and supported in designing and implementing innovations such as simulations in the health professional curriculum.

SUMMARY

Collaborative practice models that embrace simulation as a vehicle for improving patient care are timely and necessary. Interdisciplinary education is critical to delivering safe and holistic patient care.[3] Simulations that enhance collaborative practice models facilitate knowledge and appreciation of the contributions each discipline brings to the patient care arena. Moreover, understanding the expertise and abilities of each health care provider improves the likelihood that patients will receive comprehensive, quality care. Interdisciplinary simulations provide students and practicing professionals an opportunity to gather and synthesize information about the patient, about themselves, and about other members of the health care team. This valuable information then forms the basis for effective communication, critical thinking, and problem-solving that contributes to interdisciplinary collaboration and a safe practice environment.

REFERENCES

1. Morton P. Using a critical care simulation laboratory to teach students. Crit Care Nurse 1999;17(6):66–8.
2. Morton PG. Creating a laboratory that simulates the critical care environment. Crit Care Nurse 1995;16(6):76–81.
3. Institute of Medicine. Patient safety, achieving a new standard of care. Available at: Washington, DC: National Academy Press; 2003 http://www.iom.edu/CMS/3809/4629/16663.aspx. Accessed May 30, 2008.
4. Sherwood G, Thomas E, Bennett DS, et al. A teamwork model to promote patient safety in critical care. Crit Care Nurs Clin North Am 2002;14(4):333–40.
5. Fewster-Thuente L, Velsor-Friedrich B. Interdisciplinary collaboration for healthcare professionals. Nurs Adm Q 2008;32(1):40–8.
6. Baggs JG, Schmitt MH, Mushlin AL, et al. Nurse-physician collaboration and satisfaction with the decision-making process in three critical care units. Am J Crit Care 1997;6(5):393–9.
7. Griffiths M, Ibarra D, de Gonzalez A, et al. Attitudes toward physician-nurse collaboration: a cross-cultural study of male and female physicians and nurses in the United States and Mexico. Nurse Res 2001;50(2):123–8.
8. Lanning SK, Ranson SL, Willett RM. Communication skills instruction utilizing interdisciplinary peer teachers: program development and student perceptions. J Dent Educ 2008;72(2):172–82.
9. Allen KL, More FG. Clinical simulation and foundation skills: an integrated multidisciplinary approach to teaching. J Dent Educ 2004;68(4):468–74.
10. Keleher KC. Collaborative practice: characteristics, barriers, benefits, and implications for midwifery. J Nurse-Midwifery 1998;43(1):8–11.
11. Ziner-Wagler K. Asset-building and trust in interdisciplinary teamwork. Doctoral dissertation, Indiana University School of Nursing, 2006.
12. National Patient Safety Foundation. Available at: http://www.npsf.org. Accessed May 10, 2006.
13. Sexton JB, Thomas EJ, Helmreich RL. Error, stress, and teamwork in medicine and aviation: cross sectional surveys. Br Med J 2002;320(7237):745–9.
14. Fletcher GCL, McGeorge P, Flin RH, et al. Effect of a voluntary trauma system on preventable death and inappropriate care in a rural state. J Trauma 2002;54:663–70.
15. Croen LG, Hamerman D, Goetzel RZ. Interdisciplinary training for medical and nursing students: learning to collaborate in the care of geriatric patients. J Am Geriatr Soc 1984;32(1):56–61.
16. Wessell ML. Learning about interdisciplinary collaboration. J Nurs Educ 1981;20(3):39–44.
17. Williams D. Recruiting men into nursing school. Available at: Minoritynurses.com. 2008; http://www.minoritynurse.com/features/men/03-21-06e.html. Accessed May 19, 2008.
18. Zelek B, Phillips SP. Gender and power: nurses and doctors in Canada. Int J Equity Health 2003;2(1):1–5. Available at: http://www.equityhealthj.com/content/2/1/1. Accessed May 1, 2008.
19. Wear C, Keck-McNulty C. Attitudes of female nurses and female residents toward each other: a qualitative study in one U.S. teaching hospital. Association of American Medical Colleges 2004;79(4):291–301.

20. Merriam Webster online dictionary 2008. Available at: http://www.merriam-webster.com/dictionary/culture. Accessed May 1, 2008.

21. Higgins LW. Nurses' perceptions of collaborative nurse-physician transfer decisions as a predictor of patient outcomes in a medical intensive care unit. J Adv Nurs 1999;29(6):1434–43.

22. Vahey DC, Aiken LH, Sloane DM, et al. Nurse burn out and patient satisfaction. Med Care 2004;42(2):57–66.

23. Gibbons S, Adamo G, Padden D, et al. Clinical evaluation in advanced practice nursing education: using standardized patients in health assessment. J Nurs Educ 2002;41:215–21.

24. Jeffries PR. A framework for designing, implementing, and evaluating simulations used as teaching strategies in nursing. Nurs Educ Perspect 2005;2(26):96–103.

25. Cioffi J. Clinical simulations: development and validation. Nurse Educ Today 2001;21:477–86.

26. Seropian M, Brown K, Gavilanes J, et al. Simulation: not just a manikin. J Nurs Educ 2004;43(4):164–9.

27. Jeffries PR. Simulation in nursing education: from conceptualization to evaluation. New York: National League for Nursing; 2007.

28. Beaubien JM, Baker DP. The use of simulation for training teamwork skills in healthcare: how low can you go? Qual Saf Healthcare 2004;13(Suppl 1):i51–6.

29. Savoldelli GL, Naik VN, Hamstra SJ, et al. Barriers to the use of simulation-based education. Can J Anaesth 2005;52(9):944–50.

30. Seropian M. General concepts in full scale simulation: getting started. Anesth Analg 2003;97:1695–705.

31. Hammond J. Simulation in critical care and trauma education and training. Curr Opin Crit Care 2004;10(5):325–9.

32. Moyer-Childress R, Jeffries PR, Feken-Dixon C. Using collaboration to enhance the effectiveness of simulated learning in nursing education. In: Jeffries P, editor. Simulations in nursing education: from conceptualization to evaluation. New York: The National League for Nursing; 2007. p. 123–59.

33. American Heart Association and International Liaison Committee on Resuscitation. Guidelines 2000 for cardiopulmonary resuscitation and emergency cardiovascular care: an international consensus on science. Circulation 2000;102(Suppl):I1–11.

34. Awar MM, Walinsky P. Advanced cardiac life support: reviewing recommendations from the AHA guidelines. Geriatrics 2003;58(11):30–4.

35. Dager WE. Achieving optimal antiarrhythmic therapy in advanced cardiac life support. Crit Care Med 2006;34(6):1825–6.

36. Moretti MA, Cesar LAM, Nusbacher A, et al. Advanced cardiac life support training improves long-term survival from in-hospital cardiac arrest. Resuscitation 2007;72:458–65.

37. Gilligan P, Bhatarcharjee C, Knight G, et al. To lead or not to lead? Prospective controlled study of emergency nurses' provision of advanced life support team leadership. Emerg Med J 2005;22:628–32.

38. Skiba D. The millennials: have they arrived at your school of nursing? Nurs Educ Perspect 2005;26(6):370–1.

Application of the Nursing Worklife Model to the ICU Setting

Milisa Manojlovich, PhD, RN, CCRN[a],*, Heather K.S. Laschinger, PhD, RN[b]

KEYWORDS

- Work environments • Nursing leadership
- Critical care • Burnout

The ICU environment is complex and chaotic; it is no surprise that many nurses also find the ICU to be toxic. The American Association of Critical-Care Nurses (AACN) has taken the lead on addressing toxic-environment factors in their "AACN Standards for Establishing and Sustaining Healthy Work Environments."[1] Healthy work environments are satisfying: they allow nurses to be productive, give quality care, and meet personal needs.[2] Healthy work environments are those in which nurses enjoy working, remain working, and are engaged.

Sobering statistics from the US Department of Labor indicate that relief from the current nursing shortage will not come soon. For the first time in history, the supply of nurses is shrinking without administrative intervention. An aging nursing workforce, decreased enrollment in nursing schools, and rising nurse turnover rates signal that this nursing shortage differs from shortages in the past.[3] Perhaps one of the most effective personnel strategies a health care organization can take is to find ways to retain the staff it already has. Considering the research evidence linking job satisfaction and burnout to turnover,[4,5] strategies that can manipulate and configure the work environment in such a way that will reduce nurse turnover and offer nurse leaders the best opportunity to retain experienced staff are urgently needed.

The Nursing Worklife Model explains how work-environment characteristics that affect nursing practice affect nurses' lives in the workplace by contributing to or mitigating burnout.[6,7] An extension of the model was also developed and tested that demonstrated that the model could be applied to nursing job satisfaction, an outcome other than burnout.[8] The advantage to the Nursing Worklife Model is that it clearly demonstrates how various work-environment characteristics are related to each other in a systematic way. Using these characteristics, which are known to be preferred by nurses and are consistent with magnet hospital properties, will help nurse managers reduce nursing turnover by decreasing burnout and by improving job satisfaction for their staff.

The purpose of this article is to describe how the Nursing Worklife Model can be applied in the critical care setting. Within each of the five domains are multiple strategies that can be implemented to improve the practice environment for nurses.

MODEL OVERVIEW

The original Nursing Worklife Model[6] described relationships among nursing worklife factors, engagement/burnout, and nurse and patient outcomes. Five worklife factors identified by Lake[9] as characteristics of professional nursing practice environments interact with each other and affect outcomes through the burnout/engagement process. Leadership is the starting point in the model and influences the other work environment factors. Leadership has a direct effect on staff nurses' decisional involvement, staffing adequacy, and the quality of nurse–physician relationships. Leadership also has an indirect influence on the use of

[a] Division of Nursing Business and Health Systems, University of Michigan School of Nursing, 400 N. Ingalls, Room 4306, Ann Arbor, MI 48109, USA

[b] University of Western Ontario, School of Nursing, 1151 Richmond Street, London, ON, Canada N6A 5C1

* Corresponding author.

E-mail address: mmanojlo@umich.edu (M. Manojlovich).

Crit Care Nurs Clin N Am 20 (2008) 481–487
doi:10.1016/j.ccell.2008.08.004

a nursing model (versus a medical model) as the basis for care on the unit through decisional involvement and collaborative working relationships. Leadership has an impact on engagement/ burnout through staffing adequacy and the use of a nursing model of care. When staffing is insufficient to provide high-quality care, nurses are more likely to be exhausted. The use of a nursing model also directly affects staffing adequacy and personal accomplishment, suggesting that a nursing-based model of care would ensure adequate nurse staffing levels to meet the nursing needs of clients and allow nurses to provide high-quality professional nursing care. Such care, in turn, would result in greater feelings of accomplishment by the nurses and should translate into better nurse and patient outcomes.

Burnout, by definition, is a psychologic syndrome consisting of three evolving components: emotional exhaustion (characterized by feelings of fatigue, loss of concern, inadequacy, and failure); depersonalization and disengagement (characterized by a loss of emotional connection); and decreased personal accomplishment.[10] Burnout is a frequent occurrence among individuals who do "people work" such as in health care.[10] Nurses are at high risk of burnout because their emotional resources become depleted in trying to psychologically give of themselves to their patients, a situation that quickly leads to emotional exhaustion, a key hallmark of burnout.[10] In health care environments, a conflict between the desire to provide high-quality patient care and coping with workplace stress typically sets up workers to experience burnout.[11]

In the Nursing Worklife Model, exhaustion mediates the relationship of work-environment characteristics with depersonalization, which then mediates exhaustion's relationship with personal accomplishment.[6] The model has been tested in several studies, demonstrating that the unique configuration of work-environment characteristics in the model consistently contributes to burnout and other outcomes. Laschinger and Leiter[7] further showed that these characteristics were also related to patient safety outcomes, specifically, nurse-assessed adverse events. The full model is depicted in **Fig. 1**.

The five major elements of the Nursing Worklife Model represent practice environment factors under the control of nursing and are therefore amenable to improvement through nursing efforts. The following sections highlight the strategies to improve nurses' work lives through the five elements of the Nursing Worklife Model.

Nurse Manager Ability, Leadership, and Support

Nurse manager ability, leadership, and support focuses on the critical role of the nurse manager and describes key qualities that a good manager should have.[9] The prominent positioning of nursing leadership in the Nursing Worklife Model is not an accident. Nursing leadership drives the model; without it, the other domains are less effective in being able to contribute to positive nurse outcomes.

Crucial leadership characteristics that are needed are described by the AACN as authentic, transformational leadership. Transformational leadership shares elements with other leadership styles such as resonant leadership[12] and relationship-oriented leadership.[13] Although definitions of these different types of leadership vary, they are all characterized by an attention to building and sustaining relationships and the use of motivation to meet organizational goals and move toward a vision of the future.

Nursing leadership has been linked most commonly to nurse outcomes such as job satisfaction and intent to stay on the job[14] and is an important

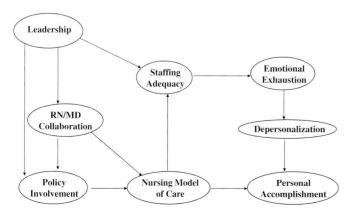

Fig. 1. Nursing Worklife Model of burnout. (*From* Leiter MP, Laschinger HKS. Relationships of work and practice environment to professional burnout: testing a causal model. Nurs Res 2006;55(2): 139; with permission.)

determinant of those two nurse outcomes. Leadership style may have a more subtle and indirect effect on nurses' intent to stay through other characteristics such as autonomy or group cohesion.[15] The relationship of nursing leadership to patient outcomes is less certain and has been the topic of research only in the past 5 years.[16]

Strategies to improve nurse manager leadership and support fall into two broad categories: interpersonal strategies and organizational strategies. Interpersonal strategies focus on having nurse managers develop interpersonal skills over time. Such strategies include managerial training to improve managers' knowledge and behaviors regarding their interpersonal, informational, and decisional roles.[15] It may be that nurse managers simply need positive reinforcement for transformational behaviors they already exhibit. One study found that many managers displayed a mix of resonant and dissonant leadership styles depending on the situation,[12] suggesting that managers already possess the skill but may need encouragement to use a resonant leadership style more consistently, which is compatible with transformational leadership.

Other strategies to improve nurse manager leadership and support can be implemented at the organizational level. One academic medical center undertook the reconfiguration of its management infrastructure, which involved putting into place administrative and clinical support for nurse managers.[17] The impetus for such large-scale change was employee dissatisfaction and the declining quality of nursing care, a tacit recognition of the influence of nursing leadership on those outcomes. Although this organizational initiative has not yet been evaluated, it is a compelling example of how a strategy targeted toward nursing leadership may make an impact with far-reaching consequences.

Staff Nurse Participation in Hospital Affairs

Staff nurse participation in hospital affairs can be thought of as an appreciation for nurses' participatory role and their valued status in the larger hospital context.[9] The Nursing Worklife Model posits that supportive nursing leadership can reduce burnout by encouraging and promoting nursing staff to participate in hospital affairs. Participating in hospital affairs offers bedside nurses an alternative and broader perspective on the health care environment and may provide opportunities to develop interpersonal skills such as participative decision making. Years of magnet hospital research have demonstrated that nurse leaders have an important role in promoting staff participation in

decision making at the bedside and in the larger organization.[18,19] Participative decision making may contribute to nurses' job satisfaction[20] and thus decrease the chance of burnout developing.

Strategic planning is a widely used organizational improvement strategy[20] and may serve as a framework for nurses to choose an area in which to become involved. Strategic planning processes may offer nurses with a wonderful opportunity to learn more about the organization and to make a substantial contribution. For example, strategic decisions often include the acquisition and divestment of resources.[20] Considering the high cost of technology and equipment upgrades, having nurses on committees to assess the purchase or upgrade of various technologies may be a cost-saving strategy for the organization and a job-satisfier for the nurses.

Other strategies for increasing nurse participation in hospital affairs include the use of "business time." In some institutions, nurses receive paid time away from the bedside to be used for quality-improvement activities or other hospital initiatives. Other mechanisms include advancement on career ladders and the development of professional practice models that can incorporate committee work to get more staff nurse participation. Some suggestions for hospital-wide committees that ICU nurses in particular may be interested in include institutional review board or ethics committees.

Finally, staff nurse participation in hospital affairs contributes to nurses' control over the context of their practice. Giving nurses the control over practice environments permits them to be involved in the design and configuration of nursing care, a necessary precursor to job satisfaction and patient outcomes.

Collegial Nurse–Physician Relations

Mutually satisfying communication and collaboration are what contribute to collegial nurse–physician relationships. According to the Nursing Worklife Model, supportive nursing leadership contributes to collegial nurse–physician relations that in turn (indirectly) reduce burnout. Physicians and nurses vary in their perspectives of what constitutes good communication.[21] Even when surveyed together, although physicians and nurses agreed that there was a direct link between disruptive physician behavior and nurses' satisfaction, the groups differed in their beliefs about responsibility, barriers to progress, and possible solutions to the problem.[22] Differing perspectives between nurses and physicians make it difficult to build consensus between the groups on how to improve nurse–physician communication.

Nurse–physician communication and nurse–physician collaboration have been the focus of nursing research in ICU settings. The classic nurse–physician communication study[23] demonstrated the importance of nursing leadership to ICU performance and patient outcomes. More recently, specific elements of nurse–physician communication were investigated for their impact on ICU patient outcomes.[24] Findings revealed that (1) the timeliness of nurse–physician communication was inversely related to the prevalence of pressure ulcers and (2) the wide variability in understanding nurse–physician communication contributed to higher ventilator-associated pneumonia rates.[24] A study of nurse–physician collaboration in ICUs showed that in the medical ICU, where there was greater collaboration between nurses and physicians, there were also improved outcomes in that ICU.[25] Although relationships between nurses and physicians may be "troubled" according to one source,[26] they are worth developing.

Collaboration has been defined as "interdependence requiring complementarity of roles."[27] This definition suggests that the disciplines of nursing and medicine offer unique contributions to patient care and that both are needed for optimal outcomes.[28] Nursing leaders may be able to facilitate nurse–physician collaboration for their nursing staff[29] by articulating the nursing perspective and its unique contribution to patient outcomes in communicating with physicians. Nurse leaders act as role models whether they are aware of it or not. When staff nurses see nursing leaders talk about nursing care issues with physicians, a tacit message that nursing issues are important is received.

There are other strategies that can help nurse leaders foster better collaboration between physicians and nursing staff. Nurse leaders who approach collaboration with physicians from a perspective of mutual trust, respect, teamwork, and open communication demonstrate to their staff the importance of these attributes to good collaboration.[27] Nursing leaders who develop these attributes and instill their importance to nursing staff will go far in promoting nurse–physician collaboration on their units.

Staffing and Resource Adequacy

Adequate staff and support resources are necessary to provide quality patient care.[9] Yet, again, strong supportive nursing leadership is needed to champion the cause of staffing and resource adequacy. This facet of the overall model is crucial to improving nurse outcomes and to mitigating burnout. High nursing workloads associated with inadequate staffing and resources contribute to burnout and to nurse turnover.

A study linking facets of the Nursing Worklife Model to nurses' job satisfaction demonstrated that the relationship between nursing leadership and staffing/resource adequacy was far weaker than that between nursing leadership and nurse participation in hospital affairs or between nursing leadership and nurse–physician collaboration.[8] These results suggest that to reduce burnout, nurse leaders need to find ways to decrease the amount of time spent on staffing issues and spend more time building collegial nurse–physician relations and promoting nurse participation in hospital affairs. Study findings echo the voices of nurse managers who said that they may spend up to 50% of their time in staffing/scheduling activities but would rather spend more time in the coaching, mentoring, and support of staff.[17]

The link between staffing and patient outcomes is strong and consistent in ICU settings.[30] A recent meta-analysis of the relationship of staffing to adverse outcomes in ICUs demonstrated that a single registered nurse (RN) full-time equivalent (FTE) increase per patient day would lead to seven fewer cases of hospital-acquired pneumonia, seven fewer cases of respiratory failure, six fewer unplanned extubations, and two fewer cardiac arrests.[30] Nursing leaders who are armed with such information are better able to make a compelling case for increasing the number of RN FTEs.

Resource adequacy is variable across inpatient units, and there are many opportunities for nurses and nursing leaders to build a business case for why a specific resource is needed. In some cases the resource may be very expensive, as in the purchase of highly technical equipment, but in other cases the resource may be relatively inexpensive. Whatever the cost of the resource, the most effective strategy is one that demonstrates how the resource improves patient or provider outcomes.

The Joint Commission's focus on patient safety affords an opportunity to link resource needs to improving some aspect of patient safety. For example, in 2008 a new patient safety goal is to improve the recognition and response to changes in a patient's condition.[31] Considering the previously discussed solid research linking staffing to better patient outcomes, nurse leaders can frame the need for hiring more nursing staff from the perspectives of improving patient safety and meeting the Joint Commission's patient safety goal.

Nursing Foundations for Quality of Care

Nursing foundations for quality of care include several factors: a pervasive nursing philosophy, a nursing model (rather than a medical model) of care delivery, and clinical nursing competence.[9] According to the Nursing Worklife Model, nurse participation in hospital affairs and collegial nurse–physician relations directly influence the extent to which nursing foundations for quality care are able to pervade a nursing unit. According to the model, the impact of nursing leadership on nursing foundations for quality care is indirect but still significant.

The most current trend in models of care delivery is actually the use of no single model of care. Recent literature suggests that implementing a single model of care delivery may or may not fit a unit's context.[32] An alternative approach is to develop a unique, setting-specific care delivery model based on an evaluation of unit-specific structure and process criteria and allocation of various provider roles.[32]

Making organizational changes are never easy, but the AACN has multiple resources to help transfigure a nursing unit. The Beacon Award for Critical Care Excellence is a program administered by the AACN. The award recognizes individual ICUs for their ability to provide exceptional care to patients and their families while at the same time providing healthy work environments for nursing staff. Units must meet 42 criteria, which are divided into 6 categories: recruitment and retention; education, training, and mentoring; evidence-based practice and research; patient outcomes; healing environment; and leadership and organizational ethics. An audit tool and step-by-step instructions, which can be used as templates to assist nurse leaders in taking the steps necessary to transform their unit, are available on the Beacon Web site (https://www.aacn.org/AACN/ICURecog.nsf/vwdoc/MainPage). Although implementing strategies such as those mentioned can seem daunting, the Nursing Worklife Model maintains that a nursing model of care in an ICU contributes to nurses' sense of personal accomplishment, providing some protection against burnout.

STRATEGIES TO DECREASE BURNOUT

Two approaches to preventing burnout are described in the literature: individual interventions and worklife interventions. Schaufeli and Buunk[33] state that individual approaches are more prevalent in the literature but argue that individual approaches place much of the blame on the individual rather than addressing sources of burnout in the work setting. Individual interventions such as cognitive-behavioral techniques that involve stress inoculation training and cognitive restructuring exercises, stress management sessions, and self-help groups are designed to increase employees' coping skills and build stronger social support networks. Van der Klink and colleagues[34] found in a meta-analysis of studies of individual approaches that cognitive-behavioral approaches were moderately effective in mitigating burnout. Relaxation training was less effective in this analysis.

Workplace interventions are advocated by several burnout theorists, although there are few reports of the effectiveness of these interventions in the literature to date. Leiter and Maslach[35] proposed a model of six areas of worklife that influence the development of burnout and are amenable to workplace interventions. They argued that when there is a mismatch among employees' expectations of workload, control, rewards, fairness, community, and values in the work setting, burnout is more likely to occur; however, there are no reports of interventions based on this model in the literature. Other workplace strategies such as job redesign, opportunities for professional development, conflict management, and effective communication training programs are recommended by Schaufeli and Buunk.[33] Supportive supervision styles and participative management approaches are also suggested by Cherniss.[36]

A combination of individual and workplace strategies is probably the most effective approach to preventing and managing burnout. Burnout prevention workshops can be integrated into hospital employee health programs, and managers can take steps to ensure that employees are empowered to accomplish their work in meaningful ways. Study results demonstrate that workplace factors that support professional nursing practice are associated with lower levels of burnout. Thus, ensuring that nursing work environments have (1) strong leadership, (2) effective collaboration among nurses and physicians, (3) staff nurse decisional involvement, (4) a strong nursing foundation of care, and (5) adequate staffing levels is an important multipronged management strategy for preventing burnout in intensive care nursing settings.

SUMMARY

In summary, the Nursing Worklife Model is a useful roadmap for thinking about how work environment factors that affect nurses' work lives interact and proceed toward staff nurse burnout. The model can best be thought of as a template to be used whenever decisions about work-environment factors need to be made. For example, nursing leaders who have many competing demands for their time will recognize that efforts to build collegial nurse–physician relations will be a better use of their time than working directly to build a nursing model of care. This is because the model demonstrates that through collegial nurse–physician relations, nurse participation in hospital affairs is likely to improve and a nursing model of care will be more likely to arise.

Nurse leaders may first want to conduct an assessment of their units to determine where initial strategies to improve nurses' work lives should be deployed. Across all five Nursing Worklife domains, however, the most compelling argument to be made is the need to reduce burnout because of its deleterious effects on nursing effectiveness and patient outcomes. In many industries, working conditions are such that employees look forward to their work and derive inspiration and great satisfaction from their jobs. The use of the Nursing Worklife Model may allow employees of the health care industry to join the ranks of their peers in other settings.

REFERENCES

1. American Association of Critical-Care Nurses. AACN standards for establishing and sustaining healthy work environments: a journey to excellence. Available at: http://aacn.org/WD/HWE/Docs/HWEStandards.pdf. Accessed June 6, 2008.
2. Kramer M, Schmalenberg C. Confirmation of a healthy work environment. Crit Care Nurse 2008;28:56–64.
3. Berliner HS, Ginzberg E. Why this hospital nursing shortage is different [see comment]. JAMA 2002;288:2742–4.
4. Laschinger HKS, Leiter MP. The Nursing Worklife Model: the role of burnout in mediating work environment's relationship with job satisfaction. In: Halbesleben JRB, editor. Handbook of stress and burnout in health care. Hauppauge (NY): Nova Science Publishers, Inc.; 2008.
5. Halm M, Peterson M, Kandels M, et al. Hospital nurse staffing and patient mortality, emotional exhaustion, and job dissatisfaction. Clin Nurse Spec 2005;19:241–51.
6. Leiter MP, Laschinger HKS. Relationships of work and practice environment to professional burnout: testing a causal model. Nurse Res 2006;55:137–46.
7. Laschinger HKS, Leiter MP. The impact of nursing work environments on patient safety outcomes: the mediating role of burnout/engagement. J Nurs Adm 2006;36:259–67.
8. Manojlovich M, Laschinger HKS. The Nursing Worklife Model: extending and refining a new theory. J Nurs Manag 2007;15:256–63.
9. Lake ET. Development of the practice environment scale of the Nursing Work Index. Res Nurs Health 2002;25:176–88.
10. Maslach C, Jackson SE. The measurement of experienced burnout. Journal of Occupational Behavior 1981;2:99–113.
11. Kalliath T, Morris R. Job satisfaction among nurses: a predictor of burnout levels. J Nurs Adm 2002;32:648–54.
12. Cummings GG, Hayduk L, Estabrooks CA. Mitigating the impact of hospital restructuring on nurses: the responsibility of emotionally intelligent leadership. Nurse Res 2005;54:2–11.
13. Anderson RA, Issel LM, McDaniel RR. Nursing homes as complex adaptive systems: relationship between management practice and resident outcomes. Nurse Res 2003;52:12–21.
14. Larrabee JH, Janney MA, Ostrow CL, et al. Predicting registered nurse job satisfaction and intent to leave. J Nurs Adm 2003;33:271–83.
15. Boyle DK, Bott MJ, Hansen HE, et al. Managers' leadership and critical care nurses' intent to stay. Am J Crit Care 1999;8:361–71.
16. Wong CA, Cummings GG. The relationship between nursing leadership and patient outcomes: a systematic review. J Nurs Manag 2007;15:508–21.
17. Dawson C, Aebersold M, Mamolen N, et al. The Michigan Leadership Model: developing a management infrastructure. J Nurs Adm 2005;35:342–9.
18. McClure ML, Poulin MA, Sovie MD, et al. Magnet hospitals: attraction and retention of professional nurses. Kansas City (MO): American Nurses' Association; 1983.
19. McClure ML, Hinshaw AS. Magnet hospitals revisited: attraction and retention of professional nurses. Washington, DC: American Nurses Publishing; 2002.
20. Kim S. Participative management and job satisfaction: lessons for management leadership. Public Adm Rev 2002;62:231–41.
21. Larson E. The impact of physician–nurse interaction on patient care. Holist Nurs Pract 1999;13:38–46.
22. Rosenstein AH, O'Daniel M. Disruptive behavior and clinical outcomes: perceptions of nurses and physicians. Am J Nurs 2005;105:54–64.
23. Shortell SM, Zimmerman JE, Rousseau DM, et al. The performance of intensive care units: does good management make a difference? Med Care 1994;32:508–25.
24. Manojlovich M, Antonakos CL, Ronis DL. ICU practice environments, RN/MD communication, and adverse patient outcomes. Am J Crit Care, in press.
25. Baggs JG, Schmitt MH, Mushlin AI, et al. Association between nurse–physician collaboration and

patient outcomes in three intensive care units [see comment]. Crit Care Med 1999;27:1991–8.

26. Greenfield LJ. Doctors and nurses: a troubled partnership. Ann Surg 1999;230:279–88.

27. Schmalenberg C, Kramer M, King CR, et al. Excellence through evidence: securing collegial/collaborative nurse–physician relationships, part 1. J Nurs Adm 2005;35:450–8.

28. Stein-Parbury J, Liaschenko J. Understanding collaboration between nurses and physicians as knowledge at work. Am J Crit Care 2007;16:470–7.

29. Boyle DK, Kochinda C. Enhancing collaborative communication of nurse and physician leadership in two intensive care units. J Nurs Adm 2004;34:60–70.

30. Kane RL, Shamliyan TA, Mueller C, et al. The association of registered nurse staffing levels and patient outcomes: systematic review and meta-analysis. Med Care 2007;45:1195–204.

31. The Joint Commission. 2008 national patient safety goals. Available at: http://www.jointcommission.org/PatientSafety/NationalPatientSafetyGoals/08_hap_npsgs.htm. Accessed June 4, 2008.

32. Deutschendorf AL. From past paradigms to future frontiers: unique care delivery models to facilitate nursing work and quality outcomes. J Nurs Adm 2003;33:52–9.

33. Schaufeli WB, Buunk BP. Burnout: an overview of 25 years of research and theorizing. In: Schabracq MJ, Winnubst JAM, Cooper CL, editors. The handbook of work and health psychology. New York: John Wiley; 2003. p. 383–425.

34. van der Klink JJL, Blonk RWB, Schene AH, et al. The benefits of interventions for work-related stress. Am J Public Health 2001;91:270–6.

35. Leiter MP, Maslach C. Areas of worklife: a structural approach to organizational predictors of job burnout. In: Cooper C, editor. Handbook of stress medicine and health. 2nd edition. London: CRC Press; 2004. p. 173–92.

36. Cherniss C. Professional burnout in human services organizations. New York: Praeger; 1980.

Bundled Redesign: Transformational Reorganization of Acute Care Delivery

Gladys M. Campbell, RN, MSN[a],*, Taya Briley, RN, BSN, JD[b]

KEYWORDS

- Models • Care delivery models
- Professional practice models • Healthy work environment
- Synergy • Acute and critical care

Given the health care challenges of cost, accessibility, quality, and safety, complicated by a severe pending workforce shortage, it is clear that the health care delivery system needs not just improvement but radical transformation. This article suggests a transformational and synergistic approach to "bundled redesign" with proposed changes in the geography of care, the systems and processes of care, the models of care delivery, and the cultures of health care organizations, such that the whole could be much greater than the sum of its parts. A proposed model for the implementation and systematic study of bundled redesign is presented with a plan for action in the State of Washington.

In 1854, Florence Nightingale was asked by Sir Sydney Herbert, the Secretary of War for the British Army, to join the Crimean War effort and organize a corps of nurses to care for soldiers who had been injured or who had fallen ill during the war effort.[1] When Nightingale reached the front of the war, she is reported to have found a 4000-bed hospital, some say 4000 hospitalized soldiers. Beginning with an effort to sanitize the hospital and to "reorganize patient care," Nightingale was able to reduce the mortality rate of soldiers from 60% to 2% within 6 months.[2] For the remarkable outcomes of her work, she was given the British "Order of Merit," and some have credited her with winning this war for the British.

Reflecting on this history, an obvious question to be asked is: How many nurses did Nightingale have to accomplish these extraordinary outcomes? One source[2] reports that Nightingale had 38 women, 18 of whom where sisters of the order. Another source[1] reports that she had 34 nurses. Clearly with a workforce so small and a task so great, she must have worked differently than today's system. In a *New York Times* article published in 1910 at the time of her death, it was reported that Sir Sydney Hubert promised Nightingale absolute authority if she would join him at the front of the Crimean War.[1] That promise of authority may be a small suggestion of the difference in the type of "resources" that she had at her disposal. Compared with acute care delivery systems of today, can one say nurses command this level of authority?

Today the war is of a different sort. Health care providers face ever expanding health care costs, increased numbers of uninsured, public outrage over medical errors, and inconsistencies in health care practices. Costs continue to escalate, emergency departments and specialty hospital areas are stressed by capacity challenges leading to routine patient diversion, and a shrinking workforce threatens access to health care for an ever expanding patient population. Providers strive to do more with less, to reduce costs, and manage the care needs of their communities. These challenges, however, lead to increased pressure on care providers and to unionization and militancy from disgruntled caregivers, both those employed by hospitals and physicians who are fast

[a] Northwest Organization of Nurse Executives, 300 Elliott Avenue West, Suite 300, Seattle, WA 98119, USA
[b] Washington State Hospital Association, 300 Elliott Avenue West, Suite 300, Seattle, WA 98119, USA
* Corresponding author.
E-mail address: gmcampbel4@aol.com (G.M. Campbell).

Crit Care Nurs Clin N Am 20 (2008) 489–498
doi:10.1016/j.ccell.2008.08.011
0899-5885/08/$ – see front matter © 2008 published by Elsevier Inc.

becoming the primary competitors to acute care hospitals. Schools of nursing, pharmacy, and others are pressed to expand their output of graduates to fill the growing need of hospitals, whereas the teachers in those schools are themselves approaching retirement and wondering how they will be replaced. There is lobbying for more state and federal funding for support of health care and for clinical education programs to shore up a system of care delivery that is severely broken.

It is clear that radical transformation in health care is needed and to achieve this requires the full investment of all members of the health care team, across all organizations. This change requires the efforts of those in leadership and direct care provision, those who are anxious for incremental measures of success, and those who have the patience for broad-based improvement and a willingness to find success over time. At this juncture, the health care system is sorely in need of improvements as significant as those achieved by Nightingale. To achieve these outcomes, the work of transformation must be approached from a broad-based perspective that is both inclusive and respectful, and innovative and creative.

WHY THE CENTRALITY OF NURSING IS CRITICAL AS ONE CONSIDERS REDESIGN IN HOSPITAL SYSTEMS

Nurses represent 54% of all health care workers who provide care to patients. Regardless of where patients are cared for, nurses are the providers that patients are most likely to interact with; spend the greatest amount of time with; and depend on for safety, comfort, and recovery.[3] Brilli and colleagues[4] in their 2001 publication from the American College of Critical Care Medicine stated that critical care nurses do the most patient assessment, evaluation, and care in the ICU. Nursing vigilance has been found to be key in the defense of patients against in-hospital errors.[5] Leaner nurse staffing patterns have been shown to increase length of stay,[6] nosocomial infections (postoperative infections, pneumonia, urinary tract infections),[7] pressure ulcers, gastrointestinal bleeding, cardiac arrest, and death from these and other causes.[8] These studies and a myriad of others show evidence that nursing care is directly linked not only to patient safety, but to patient survival. Despite this, few hospitals embrace this evidence as a call to action to build robust nursing departments or to position the voice of nursing as the leader in defining needed redesign, operational, or cultural improvements.

Given the current and predicted growth in the shortage of available registered nurses, it is imperative that the work of nursing and the environment where nursing care is delivered be structured and designed to allow nurses to make their optimal contribution to patient well-being. If the supply of nurses reaches a minimal level, those nurses who are practicing must be supported by appropriate architecture, systems and processes, models of care, and workplace cultures that allow the delivery of best nursing practice and the highest level of safety for patients.

The evidence is clear in describing the essential role that nurses play in the United States health care system. This vigilance includes the protection of patients from error, ongoing patient assessments that allow physiologic rescue before a life-threatening event occurs, comfort measures, coordination of care, and the education of patients and families as they transition from acute care to self care. The ability of nurses to provide the front-line protections and care essential to patient well-being is impacted by a host of workplace environmental factors. These factors must be transformed to mitigate the challenges faced in both the maintenance of patient safety and insurance of an effective patient care workforce.

A BIT OF HISTORICAL CONTEXT: THE ERA OF REDESIGN

Like today, the 1990s were a decade of much needed change and improvement in health care. In response to this need, models of redesign, restructure, and re-engineering were proposed in health care. The 1990 are so associated with these types of improvement efforts that redesign, restructure, and re-engineering all became the buzz words of the era. Unfortunately, the collective outcomes of this decade of redesign were so devastating for United States hospitals that providers are still recovering from the changes; just using the word "redesign" when talking to health care professionals today often gets a negative reaction. What can one learn from the 1990s to inform the transformation process needed in health care at this time?

In the 1990s providers were not only battling health care costs and a growing population of uninsured, but it was believed that major cities were soon to be over-bedded. With the complexity of the health care challenge, hospitals called in consultants to direct what was thought to be needed. The primary focus of the health care redesign driven by consultants in the 1990s was stated as "patient-focused care," but actually was cost containment. With an administrative focus on financial success and creating operational margins, consultants who could improve the bottom line were highly valued. Health care consultants were motivated to prove their ability to reduce cost and "waste" in the health care delivery system and cutting existing costs was the quickest route to financial improvement.

The largest slice of a hospital's operational cost is labor,[3] with nursing making up the largest portion of this labor cost in hospitals. One consulting group in their published work on patient-focused care stated "if we are interested in improving cost performance in hospitals, we need to begin with personnel-related costs."[9] These labor costs usually account for 50% to 60% of all expenditures.[3] Lay-offs and unrealistic productivity measures were common across the nation during this decade. After making labor cuts, hospitals struggled dramatically to cope with a smaller pool of workers, and most hired back all who had been laid off (and then some), at great expense. Although most hospitals were able to rebuild the workforce they had laid off, the hearts and minds of clinical workers had been lost to protective self-interest. Many nurses unionized, joined agencies for higher hourly salaries, or returned to work with a self-protective posture. Trust had been broken.

Physicians who suffered when health care was presented to them as a "business" decided to get a piece of the business action themselves. These physicians created powerful practice partnerships that could pressure hospitals for higher payment of services; pulled their office practices out of hospital facilities; and bought surgi-centers, out-patient specialty clinics, and intervention centers to attract the highest paying patients away from the hospital.

Possibly worst of all, an entire decade of improvement opportunity was lost in this process while health care costs continued to rise, the uninsured population grew, and tremendous challenges in patient safety and the quality of care began to be seen. Care delivery became more complex, technology more advanced and challenging, and the average length of stay in a hospital was radically reduced.

Having survived the very tumultuous 1990s providers now face head-on the unresolved issues of the past complicated by new challenges in patient safety, quality, and transparency; new business models in health care; and a workforce that is radically shrinking with each passing year. In a nation paralyzed by past failures, many believe that future success in transforming health care will come from grassroots demonstration projects, from local hospital collaboratives, and state-based initiatives rather than at the national or federal level. Transformation will be focused on the needs of patients and the ability to build a system that optimizes the contributions of professional clinicians while also eliminating waste and unnecessary cost.

REVISITING REDESIGN: GETTING IT RIGHT THIS TIME

In reviewing the literature, it is clear that an enormous amount of work on health care redesign and improvement has emerged over the past two decades. Much of this literature presents the use of scientific methods to address specific foci for redesign and quality improvement in health care. When looked at collectively, this literature seems to cluster into four distinct approach areas: (1) redesign that is focused on systems and process used in health care,[10] (2) redesign related to the physical geography or spaces and places where care is delivered,[11] (3) reorganization of models of care delivery focusing on the roles of care provision and how people in these roles work together,[12] and (4) innovation in the cultures of care delivery.[13] Each of these specific focus areas is worthy of consideration.

Systems and Processes

Hospital systems and processes are designed to support the delivery of patient care, which is the core business of the hospital. These systems within the hospital are often divided into complex collections of small, specialized work units that must interact in a coordinated fashion to meet the needs of the front-line care providers. Within each work unit there are systems or conditions that affect task complexity, redundancy, distraction, monotony, ergonomics, and role definition. Collectively, these systems and processes determine the level of whole system effectiveness and efficiency. The analysis of each specific work process and its level of complexity may indicate the degree of risk or level of efficiency delivered by the process to the larger whole of patient care. A useful framework for evaluating hospital systems and processes may use approaches from several disciplines including industrial engineering, biomechanics, and ergonomics. This framework may be organized around a specific quality improvement process like LEAN or six sigma. The purpose of system and process analysis is to improve the systems and processes of a hospital, ensure the allocation of appropriate services and resources at the point of care, allow for efficiency and effectiveness in care delivery and in the use of labor, and to ensure that process safety protects patients.

LEAN processes, six sigma analysis, time motion studies on the activities of care providers, implementation of technology, and studies of waste are all included in the transformational work done in the area of system and process improvement.

Studies have shown that documentation, medication administration, hunting and gathering or "traveling," and efforts to track down information and communicate patient and system needs consume most of a nurse's time.[14] Most nurses spend no more than 30% of their time in direct care provision and when tracking devices are used, it has been found that a nurse, on average, spends no more than 20 seconds in any one place.[14] These studies make a compelling case for the need for process improvements in traditional hospital systems.

Physical Geography

A significant health care building boom is underway with $100 billion spent on new hospital construction in the last 5 years.[15] The role of the physical environment in contributing to untoward clinical events, such as patient falls, nosocomial infections, medical errors, and staff turnover, was reported to significantly impact both the long-term outcomes and costs of providing health care in the Institute of Medicine's report on Crossing the Quality Chasm.[15] A growing body of research shows that the physical design of health care settings may unintentionally contribute to the negative outcomes of patients.[11]

Despite this knowledge, many approaches to hospital design from the 1950s and 1960s remain unchanged. Even with a dramatic reduction in hospital length of stay over the past decade, most hospitals are still designed around specialty units that assume a patient will be in the hospital long enough to be transferred multiple times during his or her single hospitalization. With an average length of stay of 4 to 5 days, many patients can barely get oriented to one unit and get to know one set of caregivers before they are transferred to another area. This movement of patients not only creates significant workload or intensity for nursing, pharmacy, patient transport, and housekeeping, but it also disrupts caregiver-patient relationships, reduces continuity of care, and creates dangerous patient "hand-offs" that are potentially unnecessary. Additionally, most hospital units outside of the ICU or maternity wards are still built as long hallways with central and distant nursing station areas. This geographic structure increases both the isolation and physical work demands on an aging and limited nursing workforce. One study cited that the average nurse walks 3 miles a shift while running these hallways. This same study found that when connected to tracking devices, some nurses moved too quickly for the tracking technology to be able to monitor them.[16]

This information suggests that acuity adaptable rooms allowing for limited transfer of patients would provide improvement in acute care delivery. Such rooms, designed in clusters or cells with optimal "sight lines" between patients and nurses, enhancing the ability to work in small cohesive teams, and where "hunting and gathering" of needed supplies, equipment, and information was minimized, would be optimal. One report by Hendrich and co-workers[17] suggested significant improvement in several areas through the use of acuity adaptable rooms. Patient transfers were reduced by 90%, medication errors were reduced by 70%, and the number of patient falls was also reduced.[17]

Beyond length of hallways and the size of patient rooms, the location of nursing stations, medication stations, and patient care supplies have been linked to positive patient outcomes, staff satisfaction, and efficiency.[18] These types of physical changes in the environment, along with privacy, air quality, color, humidity, temperature, and the removal of obstacles to work flow all enhance care delivery and efficiency. **Box 1** represents some of the design recommendations published by the National Association of Children's Hospitals and Related Institutions and seem generally applicable to all adult care environments.[11]

One additional recommendation for patient space is to abandon the long patient care corridor for "cells" of patient rooms that allow the clustering of staff, supplies, sight-lines, and communications for a group of 10 to 12 patients.

Models of Care Delivery

Models of care define the providers who are on a clinical care team, the roles of those providers,

---

Box 1
National Association of Children's Hospitals and Related Institutions recommendations for the design of care delivery environments

1. Install hand washing dispensers at each patient bedside and in all high patient volume areas
2. Install high-performance sound absorbing ceiling tiles
3. Build single family and patient rooms with adequate space for families to stay overnight
4. Increase visual access and accessibility to patients
5. Install HEPA filters in all areas housing immunocompromised patients
6. Optimize natural light in staff and patient areas
7. Install ceiling lifts to reduce workforce injuries
8. Explore the feasibility of acuity adaptable rooms to reduce patient transfers

and the systems within which they work together to care for patients. Traditional hospital models of care have nurses partnered with physicians as the leaders and coordinators of patient care delivery. In this role, nurses work with nursing assistants or unlicensed care technicians or other ancillary providers in their delivery of care. Physicians determine the patient's diagnosis, set the medical plan of care and treatment, and most generally work with the inpatient registered nurses (RNs) to assess the patient's progress toward achieving expected clinical outcomes. In this model of care, nurses often prefer an all RN staff and frequently are not skilled at the delegation of care required when the team has diversity in its membership. Care geography that takes place on a long hallway of private patient rooms leads to a "team" of nurses on a given shift that work in total isolation with little interactive assistance or consultation during care delivery.

The pending nursing shortage, which is predicted to be the most significant this country has experienced to date, may seriously impact the ability of nurses to function within this traditional and somewhat inefficient model of care. Further complicating the model is increased patient care complexity, a decreased length of stay, rapid turnover of patients, serious concerns about patient safety, and care that is often not evidence based. All factors combined necessitate that care providers function at a higher level and have sophisticated clinical, communication, and leadership skills. Despite these needs, and despite the fact that most clinical disciplines are defining the doctoral degree as the entry level into practice, most new graduate nurses are currently coming from associate degree programs. How will hospital leaders address the complexity of care requirements with lower volumes of available nurses and few nurses with higher educational levels?

Although, these questions remain unanswered, it is anticipated that masters-prepared shift-based nurse team leaders or clinical nurse leaders in small "cell" groupings of acuity adaptable rooms will work with lesser educated, less experienced RNs, new graduate RNs, nursing assistants, care technicians, and possibly others to care for an assigned group of 10 to 12 patients. The focus of this model is based on several precepts incorporated in **Box 2**.

Innovation in Cultures of Care Delivery

Organizational culture definitions are many and varied, but tend to refer to such characteristics as shared values, norms, and assumptions of the employed members of an organization. Although

---

Box 2
Factors to consider in the redesign of care delivery models

1. With higher numbers of nursing assistants, care technicians, and new graduate RNs comprising the future care team, a team leader or coordinator is needed for the oversight and support of these caregivers during their shift-to-shift in-patient care.
2. A nursing team leader or coordinator needs advanced education and skill in complex clinical care, communication, problem solving, delegation, and care coordination to meet the needs of patients with a short length of hospital stay and high degree of care complexity.
3. A clinical nurse leader may be the most appropriately prepared nurse to function as a team leader or team coordinator in the care delivery model of the future.
4. A reduction in the movement of patients through the use of acuity adaptable beds increases the opportunity for relationships with patients and families and increases the opportunity for the effective coordination of care while decreasing the labor associated with patient transfers, the risk of errors associated with patient hand-offs, and the risk of patient falls.
5. Care providers functioning as a team, lead by a clinical nurse leader, are encouraged to function in relationship with each other.
6. Accountability to the patient for the collective outcomes of nursing care provided over an episode of illness rests with the clinical nurse leader or team leader.
7. Consistency in clinical shift leadership allows the clinical nurse leader to be in closer relationship with physician partners.
8. A stronger and more consistent clinical leader for nursing care allows for a model of care with a lower number of RNs and a stronger model of delegation to unlicensed assistive personnel and to other disciplines.
9. A model of stronger and more consistent nursing clinical leadership allows nursing to have more authority and accountability for care delivery and should provide increased job satisfaction to nurses.
10. The model assumes a revised geography of care such that patients are arranged in private room "cell" groupings with care resources locally organized and nurse-patient sight-lines maximized.

---

a complex concept, organizational culture is often as simple as what employees believe to be true about their employing institution; how employees throughout an organization perceive it; and how this perception causes patterns of belief, values, and expectations. Specific characteristics of an organizational culture may include the style of management, the sense of hierarchy, decision-making authority or locus of control, communication patterns, and the perception of who has "voice" in the organization. The sense of openness or isolation and secrecy is also a characteristic of the organizational culture.

During the severe nursing shortage of the mid 1980s, the American Academy of Nursing examined the characteristics of 41 hospitals that despite this nursing shortage were successful in recruiting and retaining nurses.[13] The study of these 41 hospitals found that several organizational elements were critical to an organizational culture that retains nursing staff. These characteristics included autonomy, participative management, support for professional development, relatively high organizational status of nursing, and collaboration.[18] Additionally, multiple studies have found that measures of organizational culture are related to the incidence of adverse patient outcomes.[18] In a study that compared 39 magnet hospitals with 195 nonmagnet matched controls, the researchers found a 4.6% lower adjusted mortality for Medicare patients in magnet hospitals as compared with nonmagnet hospitals.[19] When studying inpatient units designed for the care of AIDS patients, Aiken and coworkers[20] found that positive patient outcomes were associated with magnet level organizational cultures where nurses enjoyed a greater level of responsibility for decision-making and more collegial interdisciplinary relationships. These studies are suggestive of the positive impact on staff recruitment and retention and on patient outcomes when an organizational culture supports a high level of professional decision-making and autonomy, collegiality, and respect in the workplace. Managerial structures that support professional development and participative decision-making further enhance the organizational culture.

Given the strong research supporting the positive impact on both recruitment and retention of care providers and positive clinical outcomes for patients when a positive organizational culture exists, the focus for change in this area should include eight key elements (**Box 3**).

RETHINKING REDESIGN: THE SYNERGY OF BUNDLING

Over 20 years ago, 80% of United States hospitals were reported to have inadequate nursing staff to meet the needs of patients. Some 100,000 vacancies were reported in hospital nursing positions

---

Box 3
Hospital characteristics commonly associated with a positive work culture

1. A participative decision-making structure
2. Autonomy of licensed clinicians to act within the boundaries of their license and professional expertise
3. Authority and leadership of nursing over support services
4. Effective and respectful communication structures and strong models of teamwork and collegiality
5. Adequate resources for direct care
6. Authentic and respected leadership that fosters open and transparent communications
7. Care assignment processes that foster continuity of care
8. Support for professional development

---

across the nation, with a serious impact on the day-to-day operations in those hospitals.[21] What occurred in the 1980s was the largest nursing shortage this country had seen to date. This shortage, however, pales in comparison with the 400,000 nursing vacancies that are currently predicted with the retirements of the nursing baby boomer generation.[22]

In response to the serious shortage of the 1980s, the Governing Council of the American Academy of Nursing appointed a Task Force on Nursing Practice in Hospitals, charging this task force to examine those forces or hospital characteristics that either impeded or facilitated professional nursing practice. The outcome of the work of this task force was that 10 consistent forces were identified as associated with hospitals that, in the midst of this shortage, were able consistently to attract and retain nurses.[13] This work was the beginning of the development of the magnet recognition program that is known today. Although the initial and subsequent magnet research identified first 10 "forces of magnetism" or characteristics of magnet hospitals, this number was later amended to 14 forces or characteristics similar in all magnet-designated facilities.

Hospitals who achieve magnet status are not given the option to "cherry pick" which forces they want to implement or advance, but instead are expected to commit to the demonstration of evidence that each and every one of the 14 forces is consistently in place at their hospital. This full commitment implies a synergy between forces such that the whole is greater than the sum of its parts. It is not enough to have a hospital with a shared governance model of participative management or a robust research program and support for professional development. A magnet facility must demonstrate that each and every force is strongly supported and fully developed in the organization.

The concept of the synergy of forces as a strong foundation of the magnet philosophy is equally compelling for care redesign. Although research and literature are focused on hospital geography or structure, systems and processes, models of care, or organizational culture, the question that remains is what happens if transformation in all four of these areas or "forces" is undertaken systematically over one period of time. Has the lack of traction in truly transforming the care environments come from a narrow focus that dismisses the potential simultaneous and synergistic change that could occur from interventions imposed in all four of the areas most commonly referred to in the redesign literature? By embracing the synergistic change possible through a bundled approach to redesign, nurse leaders may find a response to the nursing shortage in a redesign that allows maintenance of high-quality patient care through systems, processes, models, geography, and culture that is less labor intensive.

THE NEED FOR EVIDENCE: A PLAN FOR IMPLEMENTATION

In 2007, both the Northwest Organization of Nurse Executives (NWONE) and the Washington State Hospital Association (WSHA) were struggling with an appropriate response to the pending nursing shortage. As nursing retirements began and the number of new graduates in hospitals increased, anxiety was seen in hospital administrators, chief nursing officers, and staff nurses. Additionally, an increased focus on the impact of nursing shortages on patient and nursing outcomes from state nursing unions was seen. The rumbles of unrest over nursing shortages brought NWONE and WSHA into collaboration around the future of nursing in hospitals. To that end, they not only collaborated with the three nursing unions in the state (SEIU Healthcare, 1199NW, the United Staff Nurses Union Local 141, and the Washington State Nursing Association), but they also formed an agreement with the William D. Ruckelshaus Center of the University of Washington to help the five participating organizations jointly write legislation addressing the need for staffing committees in hospitals across the state.[23] This legislation was passed in the hopes that it would mitigate any future perceived need for state-based staffing ratios. The opposition to staffing ratios

stemmed from a belief that the true issues for nurses at the bedside went far beyond numbers and more importantly addressed the environments of care delivery.

In July of 2007, NWONE proposed a model of "bundled care redesign" to the WSHA Board of Directors at their annual retreat. This proposal defined a need for transformation in how care is delivered that went beyond narrow improvement activities or system tampering and that did not focus on the number of nurses believed needed to do business as usual in the future. The proposal boldly suggested that despite the valiant efforts of nursing schools to address the nursing shortage, there would not be enough nurses in the future to do work in the way it has been done. The proposal suggested that the important response to the nursing shortage, at the hospital level, was radically to alter how care is delivered in a way that allows nurses to work to the full limit of their licensure and to make their optimal contribution to patient care. A need to alter care geography, systems and processes of care delivery, models of care delivery, and cultures of hospital organizations was suggested as the appropriate response to the need for nursing. Given that nurses currently only spend about 30% of their time directly with patients, it seemed that one could dramatically recapture nursing care hours just by changing how nurses work in hospitals.[14] The true value and optimal contributions of nurses have not been accessed because of inadequate and seriously flawed environments, processes, models, and cultures of care, and this can be changed. From this presentation, a joint venture between NWONE and WSHA was initiated and a task force of chief executive officer and chief nurse executive partners from nine Washington State hospitals was brought together. This task force focused on writing a specific proposal for care redesign in the State of Washington over the course of three half- to full-day facilitated meetings over a 4-month period. After completion, the proposal was presented to the boards of both NWONE and WSHA and received unanimous approval from both boards. The proposal defined two implementation pathways or groups: a rapid cycle improvement pathway and a demonstration project on bundled redesign. Implementation of the project is scheduled to begin in early 2009 and fundraising is underway to be completed by the end of 2008.

The rapid-cycle improvement group gives hospitals the ability to test hospital-based redesign or improvement efforts and to share outcomes and experiences from the process. The hospitals implement one intervention at a time. As results come in, the hospital can expand the intervention to other units, abandon ineffective interventions, or try new improvement strategies. This approach recommends convening individual hospital-based focus groups with key hospital stakeholders ranging from hospital employees, such as nurses, pharmacists, technicians, and other care providers, to patients, families, and private practice physicians. These focus groups are used to inform the process on what interventions should be trialed or what improvements are needed. Specific, defined evaluation and study metrics are used to assess outcomes.

The demonstration project involves a group of hospitals working together to implement a set of uniform predetermined interventions based on the four previously noted principles of redesign. The focus of this group is to create a controlled "test" environment or incubator into which the interventions can be implemented across multiple and varied settings with outcomes measured over time. This process includes specific controls, expectations for data collection and sharing, and is overseen by a project director. The director provides onsite assistance and also ensures compliance with the parameters of the project.[24]

Hospitals participating in either approach defined by the redesign proposal have early access to knowledge of what interventions lead to measurable improvement through their participation in a protected "learning collaborative" where results and progress on redesign from both implementation approaches are shared. Through their participation, positive outcomes and learnings are shared, and the leaders involved with this project also play a role in developing, testing, and sharing local, and potentially national, best practice. Each approach allows as many hospitals as are interested to participate.

Task force members emphasized the importance of minimizing data collection burden and their desire to use measures already being collected by hospitals wherever possible. The metrics listed in this proposal are those that came from the small group work of the taskforce, but can be modified to be meaningful, yet not burdensome to the hospitals and at the discretion of the hospital boards. Metrics suggested have been categorized as quality measures, financial measures, and satisfaction measures (**Table 1**).

The level of enthusiasm and commitment to the development of this proposal and the degree to which hospital leaders are anxious to begin the implementation has been energizing. Additionally, large competitive hospitals in the region have

been willing to support the advantage of cooperation on this initiative while maintaining a collaborative spirit of competition. Planners are anxious to proceed and optimistic about what can be accomplished together.

SUMMARY

There are reasons for great pride in the United States health care system. There has been discovery and innovation in new diagnostics and new treatment regimes for disease. There is pride in the contributions of health care professionals that are too numerous to count and their commitment to the health and well-being of the nation is

Table 1
Evaluation metrics for Northwest Organization of Nurse Executives and Washington State Hospital Association bundled redesign project

Parameter	Metric
Quality	CMS measures
	Specific, defined National Quality Forum measures
	Joint Commission core measures
	Specific, defined nurse-sensitive outcome indicators
	Emergency room wait times
	Medication errors
	Volume of cardiac and respiratory arrests
	Readmission rates
Financial metrics	Registered nurse direct hours of care delivery
	Cost/unit of service
	Average daily census
	Average length of stay
	Cost/patient day
	Cost/average daily census
	Full time equivalents/adjusted occupied bed
	Net revenue
	Overtime use
	Agency nurse use
	Staff nurse turnover rates
	Staff nurse vacancy rates
Satisfaction metrics	Patient satisfaction
	Staff satisfaction
	Physician satisfaction

applauded. Unfortunately, pride may have blinded providers to the dysfunctions that have emerged in the systems and processes used to deliver care. It is necessary to take a deep and broad view of the total transformation that is now required if the triad of concerns in health care costs, patient safety and quality, and the diminishing health care workforce are to be successfully addressed. To move from thirty-seventh place in the World Health Organization's report of national health care quality[25] active steps must be taken to fix what is broken and to transform what cannot be fixed.

Those who are licensed direct care providers must remember that the license is both a gift and a statement of public trust. That license represents the trust the public has bestowed on providers to put them first, to first do no harm. There is an obligation not to support the status quo, but to do what is best for those who are called to serve. Providers are up to that task, and one can look forward to an innovative future of improvement in health care, a future that would make Florence Nightingale proud of what has been done with her legacy.

ACKNOWLEDGMENTS

The authors wish to acknowledge the strong support and assistance received from Charleen Tachibana, Immediate Past President of NWONE and CNE, Virginia Mason Medical Center; Leo Greenawalt, CEO WSHA, Seattle, WA; Swedish Hospital Medical Center, Seattle, WA; Virginia Mason Medical Center, Seattle, WA; Multicare Health System, Tacoma, WA; Seattle, VA Medical Center; Providence Everett Medical Center, Everett, WA; Peace Health Hospital, Bellingham, WA; Sunnyside Community Hospital, Tacoma, WA; Central Hospital, Wenatchee, WA; SW Washington Medical Center, Vancouver, WA.

REFERENCES

1. Archives of the New York Times, August 15, 1910. p. 7.
2. Wikipedia—free online encyclopedia, Florence Nightingale.
3. Institute of Medicine. Keeping patients safe: transforming the work environment of nurses. Washington, DC: National Academy Press; 2004.
4. Brilli R, Spevetz A, Branson R, et al. The members of the American College of Critical Care Medicine Task Force on Models of Critical Care Delivery, the Members of the American College of Critical Care Medicine Guidelines for the Definition of an Intensivists, and the Practice of Critical Care Medicine. Critical care delivery in the intensive care unit: defining clinical roles and the best practice model. Crit Care Med 2001;29(10):2007–19.
5. Rubenstein L, Chang B, Keeler E, et al. Measuring the quality of nursing surveillance activities for five diseases before and after implementation of the drug-based prospective payment system. In: Patient outcomes research: examining the effectiveness of nursing practice. Proceedings of the State of the Science conference. Bethesda, MD: NIH, National Center for Nursing Research. Washington, DC: US Government Printing; 1992.
6. Seago J. Nurse staffing, models of care delivery, and interventions. In: Shojania K, Duncan B, McDonald K, editors. Making health care safer: a critical analysis of patient safety practices, evidence report/technology assessment. No 43. Rockville (MD): AHRQ; 2001.
7. Aiken LH, Clarke SP, Sloane DM, et al. Hospital nurse staffing and patient mortality, nurse burnout, and job dissatisfaction. JAMA 2002;288(16):1987–93.
8. Needleman J, Buerhaus P, Mattke S, et al. Nurse-staffing levels and the quality of care in hospitals. N Engl J Med 2002;346(22):1715–27.
9. Lathrop JP. Restructuring health care: the patient focused paradigm, Booze-Allen Health Care. San Francisco (CA): Jossey-Bass Inc. Publishers; 1993.
10. Kaplan G, VanDawark T, Tachibana C. Virginia Mason Medical Center: seeking perfection in healthcare by applying the Toyota Production System to medicine. In: 2007 Proceedings, Nursing Leadership congress: Designing frameworks for patient safety.
11. National Association of Children's Hospitals and Related Institutions. Executive summary: evidence for innovation: transforming children's health through the physical environment, 2008.
12. Wasson JH, Godfrey MM, Nelson E, et al. Microsystems in healthcare: part 4. Planning patient-centered care. Jt Comm J Qual Saf 2003;29(5):227–37.
13. McClure M, Poulin M, Sovie M, et al. Magnet hospitals: attraction and retention of professional nurses. American Academy of Nursing Taskforce on Nursing Practice in Hospitals. Kansas City (MO): American Nursing Association; 1983.
14. Hendrich AL. Ascension health: eliminating preventable errors by 2008. In: 2007 Proceedings, Nursing Leadership Congress: Designing frameworks for patient safety.
15. Henrikson L. The role of the physical environment in crossing the quality chasm. Jt Comm J Qual Patient Saf 2007;33(Suppl):68–80.
16. 2007 Proceedings: Nursing Leadership Congress: Designing frameworks for patient safety, sponsored by McKesson, American Association of Nurse Executives, Joint Commission, National Patient Safety Foundation, Intel, Institute for Safe Medication Practices.

17. Hendrich AL, Fay J, Sorrells AK. Effects of acuity-adaptable rooms on flow of patients and delivery of care. Am J Crit Care 2004;13(1): 35–45.

18. Agency for HC Research and Quality.

19. Aiken L, Smith HL, Lake ET. Lower medicare mortality among a set of hospitals known for good nursing care. Med Care 1994;32(8):771–87.

20. Aiken L, Sloane A, Lake T, et al. Organization and outcomes of inpatient AIDS care. Med Care 1999; 37(8):760–72.

21. Aiken L. Nursing priorities for the 1980s: hospitals and nursing homes. Malaysian Journal of Nutrition 1981;81(2):324–30.

22. US Department of Health and Human Services. What is behind HRSA's projected supply, demand, and shortage of registered nurses? 2004. Available at: http://bhpr.hrsa.gov/healthworkforce/reports/behindrnprojections/4htm. Accessed July 31, 2008.

23. House Bill 3123, Washington State.

24. Northwest Organization of Nurse Executives, Washington Hospital Association, unpublished proposal on Care Redesign in the State of Washington.

25. World Health Organization. World health report 2000—health systems: improving performance. Geneva (Switzerland); Published by the World Organization. Available at: www.who.int/whr. Accessed June 21, 2000.

Index

Note: Page numbers of article titles are in **boldface** type.

Crit Care Nurs Clin N Am 20 (2008) 499–503
doi:10.1016/S0899-5885(08)00079-8

ccnursing.theclinics.com

United States Postal Service

Statement of Ownership, Management, and Circulation
(All Periodicals Publications Except Requestor Publications)

1. Publication Title	2. Publication Number	3. Filing Date
Critical Care Nursing Clinics of North America	0 0 6 - 2 7 3	9/15/08

4. Issue Frequency	5. Number of Issues Published Annually	6. Annual Subscription Price
Mar, Jun, Sep, Dec	4	$120.00

7. Complete Mailing Address of Known Office of Publication (Not printer) (Street, city, county, state, and ZIP+4)

Elsevier Inc.
360 Park Avenue South
New York, NY 10010-1710

Contact Person
Stephen Bushing

Telephone (Include area code)
215-239-3688

8. Complete Mailing Address of Headquarters or General Business Office of Publisher (Not printer)

Elsevier Inc., 360 Park Avenue South, New York, NY 10010-1710

9. Full Names and Complete Mailing Addresses of Publisher, Editor, and Managing Editor (Do not leave blank)

Publisher (Name and complete mailing address)

John Schrefer, Elsevier, Inc., 1600 John F. Kennedy Blvd. Suite 1800, Philadelphia, PA 19103-2899

Editor (Name and complete mailing address)

Alexandra Gavenda, Elsevier, Inc., 1600 John F. Kennedy Blvd. Suite 1800, Philadelphia, PA 19103-2899

Managing Editor (Name and complete mailing address)

Catherine Bewick, Elsevier, Inc., 1600 John F. Kennedy Blvd. Suite 1800, Philadelphia, PA 19103-2899

10. Owner (Do not leave blank. If the publication is owned by a corporation, give the name and address of the corporation immediately followed by the names and addresses of all stockholders owning or holding 1 percent or more of the total amount of stock. If not owned by a corporation, give the names and addresses of the individual owners. If owned by a partnership or other unincorporated firm, give its name and address as well as those of each individual owner. If the publication is published by a nonprofit organization, give its name and address.)

Full Name	Complete Mailing Address
Wholly owned subsidiary of	4520 East-West Highway
Reed/Elsevier, US holdings	Bethesda, MD 20814

11. Known Bondholders, Mortgagees, and Other Security Holders Owning or Holding 1 Percent or More of Total Amount of Bonds, Mortgages, or Other Securities. If none, check box. ☐ None

Full Name	Complete Mailing Address
N/A	

12. Tax Status (For completion by nonprofit organizations authorized to mail at nonprofit rates) (Check one)
The purpose, function, and nonprofit status of this organization and the exempt status for federal income tax purposes:
☐ Has Not Changed During Preceding 12 Months
☐ Has Changed During Preceding 12 Months (Publisher must submit explanation of change with this statement)

PS Form 3526, September 2006 (Page 1 of 3 (Instructions Page 3)) PSN 7530-01-000-9931 **PRIVACY NOTICE** See our Privacy policy in www.usps.com

---

13. Publication Title	14. Issue Date for Circulation Data Below
Critical Care Nursing Clinics of North America	September 2008

15. Extent and Nature of Circulation		Average No. Copies Each Issue During Preceding 12 Months	No. Copies of Single Issue Published Nearest to Filing Date
a. Total Number of Copies (Net press run)		1600	1500
b. Paid Circulation (By Mail and Outside the Mail)	(1) Mailed Outside-County Paid Subscriptions Stated on PS Form 3541. (Include paid distribution above nominal rate, advertiser's proof copies, and exchange copies)	770	719
	(2) Mailed In-County Paid Subscriptions Stated on PS Form 3541 (Include paid distribution above nominal rate, advertiser's proof copies, and exchange copies)		
	(3) Paid Distribution Outside the Mails Including Sales Through Dealers and Carriers, Street Vendors, Counter Sales, and Other Paid Distribution Outside USPS®	156	160
	(4) Paid Distribution by Other Classes Mailed Through the USPS (e.g. First-Class Mail®)		
c. Total Paid Distribution (Sum of 15b (1), (2), (3), and (4))	▶	926	879
d. Free or Nominal Rate Distribution (By Mail and Outside the Mail)	(1) Free or Nominal Rate Outside-County Copies Included on PS Form 3541	66	63
	(2) Free or Nominal Rate In-County Copies Included on PS Form 3541		
	(3) Free or Nominal Rate Copies Mailed at Other Classes Mailed Through the USPS (e.g. First-Class Mail)		
	(4) Free or Nominal Rate Distribution Outside the Mail (Carriers or other means)		
e. Total Free or Nominal Rate Distribution (Sum of 15d (1), (2), (3) and (4)	▶	66	63
f. Total Distribution (Sum of 15c and 15e)	▶	992	942
g. Copies not Distributed (See instructions to publishers #4 (page #3))	▶	608	558
h. Total (Sum of 15f and g)	▶	1600	1500
i. Percent Paid (15c divided by 15f times 100)		93.35%	93.31%

16. Publication of Statement of Ownership

☐ If the publication is a general publication, publication of this statement is required. Will be printed ☐ Publication not required
in the **December 2008** issue of this publication.

17. Signature and Title of Editor, Publisher, Business Manager, or Owner

[signature] — Executive Director of Subscription Services   Date September 15, 2008

I certify that all information furnished on this form is true and complete. I understand that anyone who furnishes false or misleading information on this form or who omits material or information requested on the form may be subject to criminal sanctions (including fines and imprisonment) and/or civil sanctions (including civil penalties).

PS Form 3526, September 2006 (Page 2 of 3)